feed your brain

THE COOKBOOK

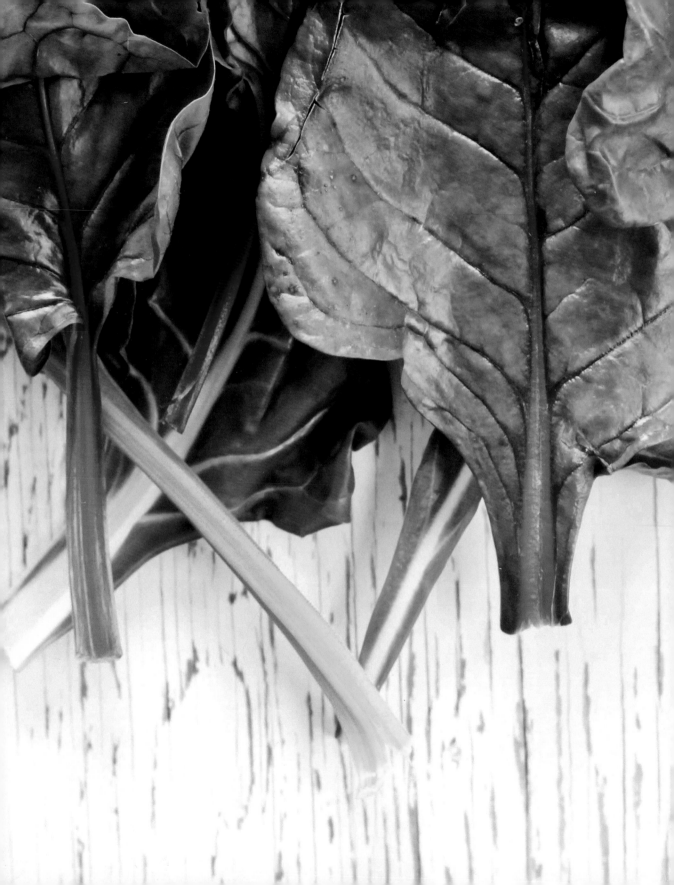

feed *your* brain

THE COOKBOOK

Recipes to Support a Lighter, Brighter You!

DELIA McCABE

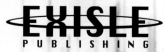

EXISLE
PUBLISHING

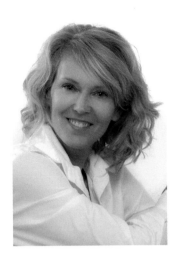

Delia McCabe has a Masters in Psychology and is completing her doctorate on the effects of certain nutrients on female stress. For the past 20 years she has combined her knowledge of the human brain with research into how food influences brain function, and a growing body of research now supports what she has seen time and again — the right diet can have a dramatic influence on our memory, moods, ability to focus and manage stress. Following the success of her first book, *Feed Your Brain*, Delia wanted to provide readers with more quick and delicious recipes to make 'brain healthy' eating even easier. You can find out more about Delia at her website www.lighterbrighteryou.life

PRAISE FOR DELIA'S FIRST BOOK:

'Wow, there is so much information in *Feed Your Brain: 7 steps to a lighter, brighter you!* on all aspects of supporting, improving and optimizing brain function. Beautifully presented, with great recipes and fabulous photos!'

Udo Erasmus, PhD., bestselling author of *Fats that Heal, Fats that Kill*

'Delia's book was a true gift. The content was enlightening, easy to read and understand, while giving practical steps to work with immediately! Applying these steps created life-changing results in my wellness, both physically and emotionally, and I find myself recommending Delia's work consistently. As a raw food chef, it's also a joy to try recipes that are delicious and nutritious, while being simple to create.'

Kisane Appleby, Realistically RAW you

'Delia's great book containing the delightful and real food, really delicious 7 step plan has literally transformed me in my retirement years into a lighter, brighter woman who is not only medication-free at almost 70, but also free to enjoy my darling little grandchildren to the max.'

Anita Earle, retired child therapist and grandmother

'My husband and I have a close history of dementia in the family and have taken a great interest in Delia's ability to transfer the science of food and how it has such a profound effect on our brains and subsequent cognition. With two growing children, we especially loved the chapters that talked about food additives as well as the sections about vitamins and minerals. Delia's book took the time to explain the types of vitamins and minerals that are in foods and what repercussions reduced vitamin/mineral intake has on our health and overall wellbeing. The kids became part of the learning so could observe not just 'what' foods are required to stay healthy but 'why' the right types of foods keep us energized and functioning optimally. They note this especially when it comes to their moods (and so do we). Thank you, Delia.'

Jen Chastre, www.nobrainr.org

'I am writing to let you know how wonderfully effective your book has been as a resource for some of my clients with mood swings, and many of my adolescent clients who suffer with depression. Your book is a fabulously in-depth resource for myself as well as for my clients.'

Robyn Rubenstein MA (Psych) MAHPRA, MAPS, MAAFT, MAJP

'*Feed Your Brain* is a powerful book that stands out from the rest. It cuts through so much "noise" out there on what to eat, with mind-blowing facts on the brain–gut connection from scientific studies, yet it is written in an understandable and easy-to-read way. The book inspired me to make changes to my diet and overall lifestyle — as a result, I feel more vitality than I ever have in my life! My thinking is sharper and clearer, and the benefits flow onto other areas of my life, such as better skin and sense of wellbeing. I gave a copy of this book to my mother, who loved it so much with its simple practical tips and recipes that she immediately ordered copies for family and friends. This should be a "go-to" book for health and nutrition, and I credit it for the positive changes it inspired me to make in my life through nutrition.'

Christine Schneider

'Although I've read numerous books on nutrition — for my family and patients' benefit — *Feed Your Brain: 7 steps to a lighter, brighter you!* is my favourite resource. It contains everything essential to maintaining a health brain (and body) laid out in an easy-to-understand, well-structured and practical way — with action plans and delicious recipes! I have several copies in my clinic for people to read whilst they wait!'

F. Tyack, Physio Fit Studio

First published 2017

Exisle Publishing Pty Ltd
PO Box 864, Chatswood, NSW 2057, Australia
226 High Street, Dunedin, 9016, New Zealand
www.exislepublishing.com

A CiP record for this book is available from the National Library of
Australia.

ISBN 978-1-925335-61-3

Designed by Tracey Gibbs
Recipe photographs by Vanessa Russell of Raspberry Creative
Produce photographs courtesy of Shutterstock
Typeset in BW Modelica
Printed in China

This book uses paper sourced under ISO 14001 guidelines from well-
managed forests and other controlled sources.

10 9 8 7 6 5 4 3 2 1

Disclaimer
This book is a general guide only and should never be a substitute for
the skill, knowledge and experience of a qualified medical professional
dealing with the facts, circumstances and symptoms of a particular case.
The nutritional, medical and health information presented in this book
is based on the research, training and professional experience of the
author, and is true and complete to the best of their knowledge. However,
this book is intended only as an informative guide; it is not intended
to replace or countermand the advice given by the reader's personal
physician. Because each person and situation is unique, the author
and the publisher urge the reader to check with a qualified healthcare
professional before using any procedure where there is a question as to
its appropriateness. The author, publisher and their distributors are not
responsible for any adverse effects or consequences resulting from the
use of the information in this book. It is the responsibility of the reader to
consult a physician or other qualified healthcare professional regarding
their personal care. This book contains references to products that may
not be available everywhere. The intent of the information provided is to
be helpful; however, there is no guarantee of results associated with the
information provided.

CONTENTS

INTRODUCTION: FEEDING YOUR HUNGRY BRAIN

There are very few people who ever think about feeding their brain — and there are even fewer books to show you how to accomplish this with enjoyment and ease. When you feed your brain what it needs to work optimally, other health challenges, such as stubborn weight gain, blood-glucose imbalances, rapid ageing, low energy levels and sleep challenges, fall away naturally. Why? Your brain is your primary survival organ, therefore it is also the hungriest and most nutrient-demanding organ that you possess. It gets first choice of the nutrients that you eat, and if you are short-changing it by eating the wrong foods and avoiding the right ones, you can't solve any health challenge. In other words, if your brain is malnourished, you can be sure that the rest of your body is going to battle to maintain health.

Fortunately, I've been researching what you need to feed your brain for over 20 years, and now you can enjoy the fabulous domino effect of great overall health by following my simple approach. This recipe book focuses on delicious foods, prepared with ease, which will improve your memory, mood, focus, concentration and learning capacity — and as fabulous side effects allow you to lose weight or maintain your ideal weight with ease, enjoy increased energy levels, sleep soundly, and generally just become a happier person. And, if you're wondering if it'll also help children reach their potential, the answer is yes! My ongoing research and 7-step approach started because of the children in my initial research group, and then I started to apply the principles I had discovered to feed my own children, my husband and of course myself. Over the years I've refined this approach to include all the latest findings related to feeding our precious brains. If you want your transition to a healthier eating pattern to be simple (and delicious), you've found the right book. Over time, I've simplified and perfected the process of making delicious 'brain' food quickly.

In this complex, competitive and often overwhelming world we have created for ourselves, maintaining optimal mental wellbeing is of great importance — in fact, it can make the difference between feeling moody and negative, with slow, unclear thinking and feeling emotionally stable and positive with quick, focused thinking. Unfortunately, this wellbeing seems to be challenging to attain and sustain, despite the attempts that many people make to find balance and wellbeing through a huge variety of healthy eating and exercise patterns. For example, the use of prescription medication — such as anti-depressants for people suffering from depression, anxiety, insomnia and social phobia; as well as medication used to manage childhood inattention, a lack of focus and behavioural challenges — has been increasing over the past few decades and there is no sign of this abating. Something is obviously wrong with how we are living, managing and experiencing our lives, and although poor food choices aren't the only reason for these challenges, improving food choices should be the foundation of all the other helpful approaches. Why? Because thinking occurs across a complex and sophisticated network of cells, chemicals, membranes and molecules within our brain, all of which require vast quantities of nutrients to function optimally.

Weighing in at about 1.3 kilograms (2.8 pounds) — a mere 2 per cent of your ideal body weight — and containing 160,000 kilometres (99,419 miles) of blood vessels, while using up a fifth of the heart's output of blood and 25 per cent of the oxygen you breathe, your brain is an amazingly active and demanding organ. The human brain is hungry for whole, nutrient-dense food with which to fuel its never-ending demand for energy and sophisticated functioning. It shouldn't, therefore, come as a surprise that psychological challenges due to nutrient deficiencies are experienced before physical ailments are noticeable. For example, moodiness, depression, an inability to focus and concentrate, and poor learning and memory capacity are psychological challenges that many people face regularly, if not daily, and simply brush off as normal or just part of ageing.

Although more and more research is being directed towards the importance of good nutrition for mental health, which I address in my book *Feed Your Brain: 7 steps to a lighter, brighter you!*, most people are still largely unaware of the impact of nutrition on brain function, probably due to the brain's performance still generally being shrouded in mystery.

This is not surprising, because it takes about seventeen years for research to filter down from academics to the general population, and possibly longer with a subject as complex as nutritional neuroscience. However, the research is accumulating: what we eat directly affects brain function. If we want to cope in this busy, complex world, which includes the multitasking and brain-draining tasks we demand of our busy brains, we need to consider this issue seriously. Unfortunately, despite all the technological advances that we enjoy today, we have less and less time to spend on preparing tasty and nutrient-dense foods while, ironically, we need them more than ever because a stressed brain uses up more nutrients than does a calm brain.

Thankfully, you do not need to swallow horrid concoctions, consume vast quantities of expensive supplements, or eat boring, bland food to support your brain's optimal health. When you keep in mind that the best food is unprocessed, and you learn how to make it tasty and enticing with the right fats, herbs and spices, you will enjoy supporting your busy brain and the benefits that this approach provides. This book is full of recipes, tips and tricks to make eating to support your brain's health a pleasure. In addition, the brain loves stimulation in the form of flavour, texture, colour and variety, so it's important to ensure that food smells, looks and tastes great. Enhancing the brain's enjoyment of eating can also help stimulate digestive juices, which in turn aids optimal digestion and absorption. When these aspects of eating are provided along with nutrient density and variety, food can be very satisfying, healthy and delicious.

Feeding your brain can be a pleasure and provide both immediate enjoyment and long-term benefits.

Over the past decade, there has been so much excitement about supplements for brain health and the introduction of exotic new superfoods, that many people have forgotten that real, easily accessible foods should form the foundation of optimal brain nutrition. Foods that are easy to find, don't travel halfway around the world from exotic destinations, have been eaten and enjoyed for millennia and contain a wealth of nutrients that are essential for both our physical and mental health need to be the cornerstone of our brain nourishment approach.

The majority of the recipes in this book are simple to prepare and allow you to mix and match according to your specific taste preference, the seasonal availability of produce and what you have in your pantry and refrigerator. As you get into the habit of preparing and eating these meals your energy levels will naturally rise and you will feel satisfied for longer after each meal. This will automatically help to stabilize your blood glucose levels, which naturally leads to fewer food cravings and can lead to weight loss over time if you need to shed weight. Feeding your brain allows your body to find your ideal weight, which for some people may mean weight gain — for example, people who have had challenges with appetite or food intolerances — or for children who are fussy eaters. In addition, your brain will get more of the nutrients it needs to function optimally, so you will be able to focus and concentrate more effectively, which leads to improved memory. On top of this, nutrient-dense foods have also been linked to improved mood. Supporting your sophisticated brain by eating the best possible nutrients is the simplest way to achieve these goals. You just need a simple understanding of what the brain needs to work effectively — and the recipes, tips and tricks in this book will guide you.

Feeding your brain what it needs to function optimally is not challenging, although it does take some planning and forethought. But rest assured that the benefits far outweigh the changes required — and they last a lifetime.

We need to use the knowledge we have about what our brains require to function optimally to support their wellbeing and health into old age. In order to feel the benefit of a fully functioning and healthy brain — which can impact your ability to live your best life and age well — you must take your food choices seriously and make good decisions.

These decisions can do two things: they can either support us in fulfilling our dreams and goals, or they can undermine us, because what we choose to eat can support our thinking, the choices and decisions we make, how we manage challenges and adversity and, ultimately, the quality of our lives. Enjoy living your best life by feeding your brain!

SUMMARY OF THE 7 STEPS TO A LIGHTER, BRIGHTER YOU!

In *Feed Your Brain: 7 steps to a lighter, brighter you!* I delve deeply into the science behind how feeding your brain leads to improved mental wellbeing, which includes the ability to improve focus and concentration, naturally improve learning and memory capacity as well as mood, and weight loss over time if you need to lose weight. Here is a quick summary of those seven steps.

1) Sweat, sleep, sex and stress — what they mean to your brain

More and more research is revealing that when we take care of our bodies through exercise, when we reduce and manage our stress levels and surround ourselves with loving and supportive relationships, we help our brain to stay healthy for as long as possible. Add great sleep and the pleasure of sex to this mix, and our brains have the opportunity to work efficiently, and provide us with the support we need to remain calm, happy and productive in our busy lives. Our brains respond to these positive activities, and the reduction of stress, by becoming more robust at the cellular level, thereby enhancing neuronal functioning.

What you need to focus on is becoming more physically active, reducing your stress levels naturally and improving your relationships, along with getting more restorative sleep and boosting your sex life.

2) What food intolerances do to your brain

Specific foods are more likely to cause a brain reaction — and addiction — than others, and knowing which ones they are, and removing them from our diet, can improve our brain function. In addition, optimal digestive health is critically important for our busy brains and by ensuring ideal digestion and absorption are maintained, we can improve our brain's ability to function optimally.

What you need to focus on is removing the foods that you may be intolerant to, such as gluten and/or dairy, among others, and improving gut function, both of which directly impact mental health.

3) Why food additives are bad for your brain

Modern food processing uses a vast quantity of additives to ensure shelf stability, and also removes compounds, such as fibre, which are important for optimal health. Unfortunately, the majority of the additives used in processed food are not tested in combination, so their safety is questionable, especially with regard to brain function. In addition, a number of additives pose a direct threat to brain cells, and removing them from our diet is critically important for brain health. Heavy metals and other toxic compounds found in many household cleaning products and pesticides also pose a threat to our delicate brains.

What you need to focus on is eating mostly whole, unprocessed foods that haven't visited a factory before you buy them, such as colourful fresh produce and whole, gluten-free grains and legumes; making your own salad dressings and sauces; and avoiding additives in the minimally processed foods you might eat, such as rice cakes or crackers.

4) The vitamins and minerals your brain needs

Vitamins and minerals are crucially important for optimum brain health because the brain uses them to generate energy, make neurotransmitters, and ensure membrane flexibility and permeability, among many other activities. These nutrients have specific roles to play in the brain, and modern diets, as well as very restrictive diets, can irreparably compromise brain development, growth and maintenance. Antioxidants in whole, unprocessed foods also support great brain health by quenching free-radical activity and the dangers it poses to brain health. In addition, pure, clean water is required to ensure optimal brain function, because dehydration has a direct and immediate effect on the brain's ability to function.

What you need to focus on is eating a large variety of seasonal, colourful fresh fruit and vegetables as well as sprouts, and whole, gluten-free grains, legumes and nuts and seeds, while supplementing wisely with nutrients, according to your specific needs.

5) Protein and communication in your brain

Neurotransmitters are tiny compounds that brain cells use to communicate with each other; they are made from the building blocks of protein, amino acids, along with other nutrients, that our diets need to provide. Mood-altering substances, from coffee to antidepressants, impact these neurotransmitters. Although many people believe that animal products and protein powders are the best sources of protein, they may come with risks to optimum brain function. Poor digestion and inadequate liver function also impact the body's ability to make these messengers with ease.

What you need to focus on is eating a variety of gluten-free grains, such as quinoa and millet, along with legumes, sprouts, nuts and seeds. If you choose to eat animal products they should be organic, and all animal flesh should be both organic and grass fed. Most fish in the ocean live in contaminated seawater, so wild-caught fish is the best option, but it should not be relied on to supply the brain's requirement for protein.

6) Stable energy for your brain

Carbohydrates are the brain's primary source of fuel, and although there are different forms of carbohydrates, the brain prefers unprocessed, nutrient-dense, high-fibre forms rather than quick-release types that negatively impact blood glucose. Coffee provides a temporary solution to a tired brain, artificial sweeteners come with their own dangers, while refined sugars contribute to general physical and cognitive ageing. Ensuring all meals (and snacks) contain unrefined carbohydrates will deliver a steady supply of glucose to keep the brain fuelled, along with the ability to sustain an even mood, and focused thinking.

What you need to focus on is whole, unprocessed, fibre-rich carbohydrates such as leafy greens, brassicas (cruciferous vegetables), coloured root vegetables, gluten-free grains and legumes along with fresh fruit and berries.

7) The foundation fats for your brain

Fats and oils are one of the most misunderstood topics in nutrition, and with the dry weight of the brain being 60 per cent fat, it is a very important issue to grasp fully. Although the body can make both saturated and monounsaturated fats, it cannot make polyunsaturated fats, which comprise 20–25 per cent of the brain's 60 per cent fat. Unfortunately most people eat too many damaged fats and are therefore not getting enough of the right fats to ensure their brain is working optimally. Additionally, cooking with the wrong fats leads to the consumption of more damaged fats. Research has shown that the consumption of the right fats can improve brain development and overall function.

What you need to focus on is cold-pressed, organic oils that are stored in dark glass bottles. Coconut oil and butter are good sources of saturated fats; extra-virgin, single-origin olive oil is a good choice of monounsaturated fats; and a balanced blend of omega-3 and omega-6 essential fats (EFAs) is best as the source of polyunsaturated fats.

Top brain foods

Naturally, any of the minimally processed foods included in the recipes in this book follow these seven steps and therefore include organic and additive-free products, along with cold-pressed oils, and are free of salt and refined or artificial sugars. Here is a list of the top brain foods, all of which are made up of whole, unprocessed (except for the chocolate) natural foods that are nutrient-dense and supply our busy brains with the building blocks for optimal cognitive health and wellbeing.

- Colourful foods — green leaves, red and purple berries, fruit and vegetables, orange fruit and vegetables, brassicas (cruciferous vegetables)
- A wide variety of nuts and seeds, including organic cold-pressed nut and seed oils as well as oily fruit such as avocados and olives
- Whole, unprocessed, gluten-free grains and legumes
- Spices and herbs, such as turmeric, ginger, coriander (cilantro), basil and other green herbs
- Dark chocolate (at least 70 per cent)
- Sprouts
- Organic superfoods, such as goji, camu camu and maqui berries and minimally processed superfood powders, such as barley grass and acai powder
- Organic, grass-fed animal products in moderation

EVOLUTION VERSUS REVOLUTION

No one likes to have change forced on them, especially with regard to their eating habits. When you make drastic changes to your lifestyle it is easy to fall back into old patterns fairly quickly. However, if you make changes slowly, and manage to stick to these new habits, you will have far greater success. Evolution is far more successful than revolution — and longer lasting! I have often advised parents not to say a word to their children when they plan to change the family's foods in order to improve overall health. By simply including a few new dishes and some more raw veggies, change can be slow but steady, especially when the new foods taste good. Start by making a healthy treat or a delicious salad dressing rather than changing your whole dietary approach, and you will be much more likely to have a receptive family. And remember that everyone, not just children, sees better than they hear, so being an example is always a better idea than being a lecturer.

HOW TO USE THIS RECIPE BOOK

Very few people have enough time to spend leisurely hours in the kitchen preparing elaborate meals for their loved ones. Fortunately there are a few simple tricks (and recipes) that you can quickly learn to make preparing tasty meals easier — and healthier. Keeping your pantry and freezer stocked with foods that you can easily use is a wonderful start. Then, purchasing (or even better, growing) fresh, seasonal produce and herbs

Gather, prepare and eat food with purpose and intent.

every week ensures great meals are very simple to prepare. If you also keep a stash of the spices that make up the blends in this book, you can add flavour to your meals in a few seconds. Many of these recipes will become staples in your home, as they have become in mine. This recipe book contains only plant-based foods, and I encourage meat-eaters to experiment with these meals to add more nutrient-dense foods aimed at optimal brain health to their daily food choices.

I want you to always look at your meal and ask yourself this question: 'What can I add to increase the nutrient density and hence the brain-nourishing aspect of this meal?' You can add pesto, salad dressing, a sprinkle of cooked quinoa, nuts, seeds or herbs, to ensure that each meal is packed with nutrients to keep your busy brain nourished and satisfied.

SIMPLICITY, TIME CONSTRAINTS AND PREPARATION METHODS

In the interests of simplicity and saving time, I have made the recipe measurements as uncomplicated as possible. Most busy people do not have the time to haul scales out of hiding — if they have them — to measure ingredients and, more importantly, the success or failure of 99 per cent of the recipes in this book does not hang on a thread. A few of the recipes require a scale to measure — for example, chocolate, and everyone will make the effort for that!

KITCHEN TOOLS TO MAKE LIFE SIMPLER

Most food preparation can be done by hand, but there are occasions — you might want to achieve a particular texture, or simply save time and effort — when an electric machine will come in very handy. It can help you prepare food quickly, make it tastier, prettier and more exciting and introduce different food textures to a meal. Selecting kitchen appliances is an individual matter — it depends on what you can get the most use out of, what you already have and, of course, what you can afford. The varieties of recipes that you can master with these appliances will also ensure that food preparation becomes more of an adventure than an odious task. (See the resources guide on page 228 for details of kitchen appliances.)

The following kitchen appliances will make your life easier when preparing food.
- A couple of good chef's knives — small and large.
- Measuring spoons and cups.
- A sturdy, solid chopping board.
- A small and large colander as well as a few sieves.
- A good food processor, with attachments that allow you to grate, chop and mix.
- A powerful blender that can blend food to a smooth pulp or cream. You can get an attachment for the blender that can even grind wheat, rice and other legumes into flour. Although I use a powerful blender for many of the recipes in this book, if you soak the nuts (and rice and legumes, for some recipes) you can use a powerful food processor in its place. However, for the creamiest, smoothest results for many of the dressings and raw desserts, I recommend a powerful blender.

- A mandolin, with a variety of blades to grate and julienne fresh produce.

- A good set of pots, with tight-fitting lids, so that you use very little water while cooking or lightly steaming your vegetables, and therefore lose fewer nutrients.

- A slow cooker.

- A dehydrator. (This can help you dry extra fruit and vegetables when you have the opportunity to purchase — or pick — a large quantity of produce during its peak season. However, you can also use your oven set to the lowest setting, to dehydrate produce.)

- A variety of freezer- and oven-safe glass containers with tight-fitting lids (use these to store foods in the freezer and refrigerator and as baking dishes too).

- A timer. (If your oven doesn't have a timer — or you haven't learned how to use it — start using the one on your smart phone or purchase a simple timer from any kitchen store.)

- A non-stick frying pan. There is a lot of controversy over whether regular non-stick frying pans contain compounds that leach into food when heated, and I therefore err on the side of caution, and only use a ceramic frying pan. (See resources on page 228 for more detail.)

- A rice cooker doesn't only cook rice; it can also cook quinoa and millet, making the cooking of these grains much simpler than stovetop cooking.

EAT SEASONALLY

Fresh, locally grown produce naturally contains more nutrients than produce that has been in storage or travelled vast distances to get to your plate, so, where possible, eat seasonally. You will find that the recipes in this book generally reflect seasonal availability, although I do make an exception for avocados, because they are such a wonderful addition to brain-friendly food, and I'm fortunate to live in an area where they are available for most of the year. Naturally, fresh fruit that is frozen, such as berries and mangoes, does find its way into my smoothies and salad dressings.

PREPARING FRUIT AND VEGETABLES

When choosing fruit and vegetables, I select organic produce, which is generally small–medium sized. When preparing your fruit and vegetables, keep the following points in mind.

- Wash fresh produce before cooking, but don't soak it — unless it's very dirty — because this draws out nutrients.

- Cut produce only when you are ready to use it, because exposure to the air causes loss of nutrients. Additionally, vegetables that retain their skin are more nutritious, with higher nutrient and fibre content (many nutrients are found just under the skin, which is another reason to choose organic).

- Use very little water when cooking, because nutrients are leached out with this cooking method. Simply steaming or lightly blanching are healthier options. Boiled vegetables lose 20-50 per cent of their B vitamins, 50 per cent of their vitamin C and 20 per cent of their mineral content. Simply ensure that you have a tight-fitting lid and only cook vegetables until they are crunchy — not soft and limp.

- Lightly roasting vegetables is another simple and tasty method of preparing fresh produce.

> **To cube** — cut produce into about 1-centimetre/½-inch pieces
>
> **To dice** — cut produce into about ½-centimetre/¼-inch pieces
>
> **To mince** — place in food processor on low speed
>
> **To grate** — use food processor grating attachment
>
> **To slice** — either cut very thinly or thickly, depending on recipe requirements; you can also cut diagonally as a change

A goal without a plan is just a wish.

ANTOINE DE SAINT-EXUPÉRY

OUR FOOD CHOICES AFFECT OUR PLANET

Organic food is grown without artificial fertilizers, pesticides or herbicides. Natural fertilizers and composts along with crop rotation are used, which ensures healthy soil resulting in vibrant plants packed full of nutrients. The average conventionally grown apple has between 20 and 30 artificial poisons on its skin, whereas organic produce is not covered in these poisonous cocktails. Fresh, organic produce contains about 50 per cent more vitamins, minerals, enzymes and other phyto-nutrients than conventionally farmed produce.

All factory-farmed animals are fed a cocktail of drugs on a daily basis, many of which have not been tested for their effects on our health, and which we consume when we eat them and products produced from them, such as cheese, butter and eggs. Conventional farming is also destructive in other ways: the health of farm workers using pesticides is compromised, soil often becomes eroded due to poor management, the waterways become contaminated with chemicals and the creatures living in the rivers and the sea are affected, and the forests being destroyed for mono-crops such as palm oil are also injured and lose their homes. In addition, the impact of genetically modified organisms (GMOs) is still being debated, and no long-term human-safety tests have been conducted on the consumption of these foods, nor have there been any thorough environmental assessments done to ascertain what happens when these plants are released into our ecosystem. Therefore, choosing to eat organic produce has a very beneficial ripple effect on our planet, and starts with a simple decision to feed yourself and your family the best whole, nutrient-dense and uncontaminated food you can find.

PLANNING – TO FEED YOUR BRAIN

Success in any endeavour depends on a good plan that is well executed. Planning and preparing brain-nourishing food is no exception, and using the tips and tricks below will give you a head start to accomplish this with ease. The aim is to make preparing delicious meals simple, effortless and fast by using your freezer and refrigerator cleverly. I've used these tips and tricks in my kitchen for many years, and now they are well-established habits that serve me and my family every day. You can use them with ease too, and before you know it they will be just as helpful as they are for me.

USE YOUR FREEZER AS A TIME-SAVING AND NUTRIENT-PRESERVATION DEVICE

Although most of the meals I prepare use fresh, seasonal produce, I also live in the real world, and use my freezer to maximize the variety, flavour and nutrient density of my meals throughout the year.

Here are my favourite ways of using my freezer to store and preserve fresh produce when it is in season (remembering that you need to use freezer-proof glass containers).

- Freezing extra fruit, such as mangoes and strawberries, when the season brings you an abundance of them, allows you to make memorable smoothies, desserts and breakfasts in a few minutes. Frozen, over-ripe bananas produce the most wonderful ice-cream and 'milks' to pour over breakfast cereal, as well as adding flavour and texture to smoothies.

- When tomatoes are in season, you can skin a few extra and store them in the freezer for last-minute sauces and soups.

- When capsicums (bell peppers) are in season I roast quite a few and then freeze them, to use later for hummus, soup and salad dressings.

- Wash herbs and remove leaves from stems. Grind the leaves in a blender with some olive oil and store the mixture in small glass containers to use for salad dressings, sauces and soups.

- Freeze a whole lemon and grate it over a salad (with a dollop of olive oil and a sprinkle of herb salt) for a quick burst of sunshine when you don't have another dressing on hand.

- Freeze fresh ginger roots and grate the frozen root into dishes as you prepare them.

- Freeze lemon juice and rind in small glass containers to use in salad dressings when lemons are not in season or you've run out of fresh lemons.

- Freeze orange rind in small glass containers to use in curries and sprinkle over salads.

- Freeze coconut cream and milk in small glass containers to use in cold smoothies and 'milks'.

- Freeze fresh pesto for when fresh herbs aren't plentiful.

- Freeze coconut milk in an ice-cube tray and then empty into a large glass container with a lid for use in smoothies and cold plant-based milk drinks.

WEEKEND PREPARATION

Here are my favourite plan-ahead-for-a-busy-week activities that I usually do on a Sunday. First I head to my local organic market for fresh fruit, vegetables, herbs and sprouts and then ...

> Be sure to store your nuts and seeds in the fridge or freezer because the precious oils in these compact and nutritious foods easily go rancid when exposed to light and heat over time.

- Soak legumes and nuts. (See pages 25 and 26, where soaking and cooking legumes and soaking and activating nuts are explained.) These two plan-ahead tasks actually start on Saturday night.

- Remove the rind of three or four lemons then squeeze them, storing both in a glass container for use during the week. (I only use organic lemons and oranges, but I still scrub the skin well before I remove the rind. Do not use the rind of conventionally grown citrus fruit, because pesticides accumulate in the skin, and even a good scrub or the use of products advertised as pesticide-removers, may not remove them all.)

- Soak brown-skinned nuts to make activated nuts on Monday evening. Rinse and drain very well before dehydrating the next morning or freeze for use in smoothies. (See page 19 for an explanation of why soaking nuts is important.)

- Steam a few beetroot (beets), cool and remove skin and then slice thinly and toss with the juice and rind of a lemon, olive oil and herb salt to use during the week.

- In a small (1½ cup capacity) glass container, soak 4 tablespoons of chia seeds in either:
  - 1¼ cups fresh orange juice and rind
  - 1¼ cups pomegranate juice
  - 1¼ cups coconut milk and 1 drop vanilla
  - 1¼ cups coconut milk, 1 tablespoon of raw cacao powder and 1 drop vanilla (which also makes lovely chia 'pudding')
  - 1¼ cups blueberry juice with 1 teaspoon acai powder.
- Wash herbs well, especially fresh coriander (cilantro), which often gets sand stuck in its roots, and wrap in paper towels and pack into plastic bags, removing the air from them, for use during the week. Also, make pesto using fresh herbs — see pages 72 and 73.
- Prepare salad veggies such as green beans, snow peas (mangetout), lettuce, leeks, spring onions (shallots, scallions), etc. by trimming off the ends or washing them well and storing in a large glass container, with a paper towel to catch water and keep them dry.
- Slice a red onion and add it to a glass dish with the juice and rind of half a lemon, and top up with olive oil — use as garnish and tossed into salads.
- Slice sun-dried tomatoes into slivers and add to a glass dish with olive oil and Italian herbs to use on salads and tossed through rice and quinoa or millet dishes (see pages 165—173).
- Grate a beetroot (beet) and add it to a glass dish, then cover with the juice and rind of a lemon, olive oil and a pinch of herb salt — mix well and use to top salads or stir through rice, quinoa or millet for children (or adults who still love pink food!).
- Cook 1–2 cups of quinoa (see page 29) to use in salads (see pages 89—117), as a breakfast dish (see page 41) or simply to sprinkle over salads to add extra nutrients.
- Scrub a few sweet potatoes well and cut into cubes, then toss in 1 tablespoon of coconut oil and herb salt and 2 teaspoons each of ground cumin, coriander, turmeric and ginger and bake at 120°C/250°F until cooked through and soft. Serve with salad for dinner (see page 102) or keep for use during the week. At the same time, roast a head of garlic (see page 70) to use in a salad dressing during the week.

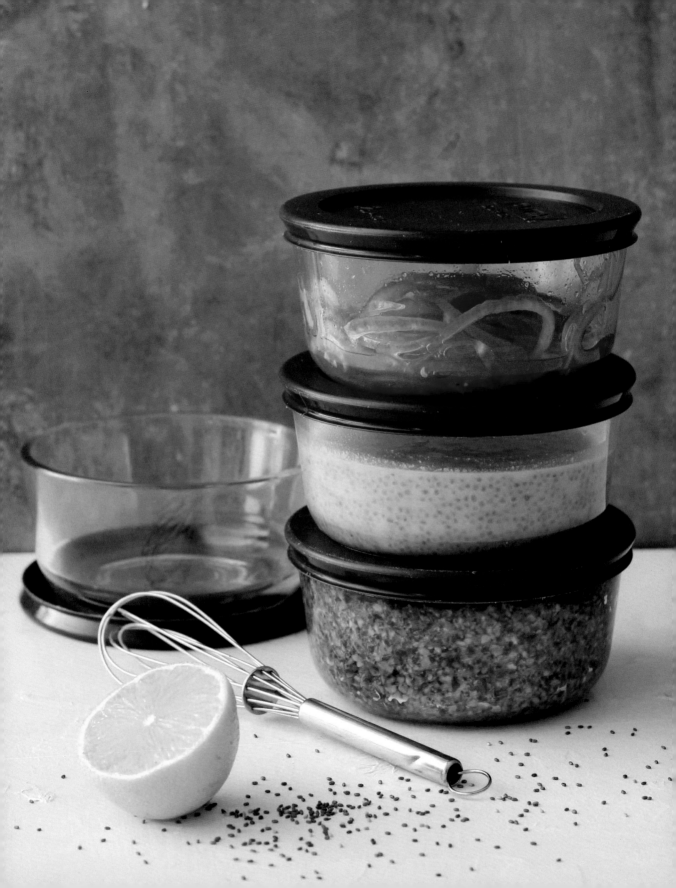

- Instant smoothie packs: In a glass container, combine everything that you would add to a smoothie except for the liquid (such as coconut milk, coconut water, almond or rice milk). Here are some of my favourite variations:
    - Banana, pecan and carob
    - Banana and peanut butter
    - Banana, raw cacao, walnut and vanilla
    - Blueberry and almond
    - Cherry, cashew and raw cacao
    - Raspberry and brazil nut
    - Mango, pineapple and macadamia

LEFTOVERS

Leftovers from most of the recipes in this book can easily be used for lunch the next day. For example, you can add an avocado and some nuts and seeds to any leftover salad. Bean and lentil stews are also great the next day. This removes the dilemma over what foods to purchase during the day, when your busy brain needs support for a hectic afternoon, and also saves you money. I always make extra salad with my evening meal so that I have some to use the next day. This will easily become a habit for you too.

SUMMARY

The aim of these tips, along with the recipes in this book, is to enable you to prepare delicious, simple, healthy, nutrient-dense and brain-healthy meals and snacks with minimum fuss and time. You can mix and match most of the recipes with different dressings and seasonal vegetables, and add toppings according to the variations described beneath most recipes, so you will end up creating new meals and delicious combinations if you simply trust yourself to do so and experiment a little with new flavours, textures and tastes. My mix-and-match approach increases nutrient density, variety and flavour with ease and also saves loads of time. The added bonus is that you become more creative with food and start to trust your instincts for which foods complement each other.

FAQS

IS IT MORE EXPENSIVE TO EAT THIS WAY?

If you buy nuts, seeds, legumes and grains in bulk and store them in your freezer you can save money while keeping them fresh, which is very important, especially in the case of nuts and seeds that quickly go rancid. Focusing on seasonal produce will also keep costs lower versus buying expensive out-of-season produce. Try growing lettuces and herbs in your back garden or on your windowsill. Initially, you may spend a little more money stocking your pantry with nuts, seeds and good-quality oils, but as you naturally spend less on processed foods — and doctors' bills — you will find that it isn't significantly more expensive to eat with brain health in mind.

WHY SHOULD I SOAK NUTS AND SEEDS?

Soaking all nuts and seeds before using them is a good idea, but soaking those that have a brown skin is especially important, if you want to maximize nutrient absorption. The brown skin that covers many nuts contains an enzyme inhibitor meant to stop insects and worms from eating the nut before it germinates. Unfortunately, this bitter-tasting enzyme can also make it difficult for us to digest these precious foods optimally, which is why soaking these nuts can make the digestion, and therefore the absorption of the nutrients in these nuts, much more efficient. In addition, soaking them also releases vital nutrients that are required by the nut to germinate. In other words, soaking them does what the rain would do: it prepares them to germinate by increasing their vital energy. I use activated brown-skinned nuts in all my recipes. See page 25 for notes on soaking nuts.

WHY SHOULD I SOAK LEGUMES AND GRAINS BEFORE COOKING THEM?

Legumes and grains (including quinoa, which is technically not a grain), along with nuts and seeds, contain phytic acid, which binds with other minerals such as calcium, magnesium, iron and zinc, rendering these minerals unavailable in the process of digesting and absorbing nutrients from these foods. Phytic acid also inhibits digestive enzymes. Soaking legumes and grains (and nuts and seeds) removes some of the phytic acid, and cooking them further reduces this compound, which means we can use these minerals, both in these grains and in the other foods that we are eating them with. See pages 25–6 for notes on soaking legumes and grains.

IS RAW FOOD HEALTHIER THAN COOKED FOOD?

Research clearly shows that a combination of raw and cooked foods provides the best health benefits, for a number of reasons. Digestion is easier with cooked food, because cellulose (fibre) is softened, and also because some phytochemicals are released though cooking that can't be released otherwise. Raw food offers enzymes and other nutrients that are decreased through cooking. Eating and digesting only raw food is energy intensive and means that eating has to occur every few hours to keep nutrient supply optimal. An increase in the volume of food that occurs with raw food intake, versus an increase in calories, which cooked food provides, is a reason that many people who want to lose weight choose to eat predominantly raw foods. Research into brain development indicates that discovering the ability to cook our food helped our brains develop because we then had access to concentrated forms of energy and had time to spend on creative pursuits besides continuously foraging for food. The brain is the most demanding organ in terms of energy requirements, using 22 times the amount of energy versus the equivalent piece of muscle tissue, so eating both raw and cooked food may be the best solution for our busy brains.

IS ANIMAL PROTEIN BETTER FOR YOU THAN PLANT PROTEIN?

Many people are still under the impression that only animal protein is useful as a source of 'complete' protein. Plant foods do contain a mixture of the foundations of protein, namely amino acids, and therefore, as long as a large variety of these foods is eaten over a period of a few days, plant forms of protein can provide us with the full complement of amino acids with which to thrive. Therefore, food combining daily to make a whole protein using a variety of plant forms is no longer considered essential, although it is interesting to note that many plant foods are traditionally eaten together, which results in a full amino-acid complement from the meal, for example, beans and corn chips, rice and beans, and baked beans on toast. Plant foods are also full of fibre and contain many other essential nutrients that animal products do not. Non-organic animal foods contain pesticides, hormones and antibiotics, all of which pose specific threats to our delicate brain tissue. However, feel free to add organic, grass-fed animal products to the recipes in this book, although you may want to limit this to a few times a week rather than every day.

Carbohydrate and protein sources and uses

Carbohydrates (GF) and Protein	Uses
Quinoa	To replace rice, flour, flakes, in salads and stir-fries, crackers
Millet	To replace rice, flour, flakes, in salads, stir-fries
Rice (brown, basmati, jasmine, wild, etcetera)	To be used as grains, noodles, flour, in salads, as a cracker topping
Sweet potato/Kumara	Serve as 'chips', mashed, baked, stuffed, in soup, in curries, roasted
Corn	Serve on the cob, frozen, in salads, with polenta (soft, hard, in muffins), in tortillas, flour
Buckwheat	Serve with noodles, in salads, muesli, as a smoothie topping
Peas	Serve in salads, stews, stir-fries, soups
Sprouted seeds	Serve in salads, stir-fries, as a cracker topping
Seeds	Serve in salads, pesto, in smoothies and as toppings, to make 'milks'
Nuts	Serve in salads, pesto, as a snack, in cookies, muffins, in smoothies and as a topping, to make 'milks,' ice-cream and cream
Legumes (beans and lentils)	Serve in salads, stews, dips

Plant-based food combinations to produce full amino acid (protein) complement in one meal

Food group	Limiting amino acids	Combine with
Legumes (lentils, beans, chickpeas/garbanzo beans)	tryptophan, methionine	Grains, nuts/seeds (e.g. lentil/bean soup or chickpea/garbanzo bean salad with cornbread)
Grains (rice, wheat, rye, barley, oats, corn)	lysine, isoleucine, threonine	Legumes (for example bean nachos with tortillas or corn chips)
Nuts/seeds (almonds, Brazils, cashews, hazelnuts, macadamias, etcetera, and sesame, sunflower, pumpkin seeds/pepitas, etcetera)	lysine, isoleucine	Legumes (for example kidney bean soup or four-bean salad with nut pesto or gluten-free cereal with nut milk)

Note: Vitamin B12 and possibly iron are required in supplement form when following a vegetarian or vegan diet and are critically important for both brain development and functioning throughout life.

WHY USE COCONUT OIL, CREAM AND MILK IN RECIPES VERSUS OLIVE OIL AND OTHER SHELF-STABLE OILS?

As I have discussed, the dry weight of our brain is 60 per cent fat, with 20–25 per cent of that fat being polyunsaturated fat and the other 75–80 per cent being saturated fat. We now know that the fats contained in coconuts are healthy saturated fats, which contain antibacterial, antifungal and antiviral benefits due to the presence of medium chain triglycerides (MCTs). These special fats also provide a direct source of fuel for the brain. In addition, these saturated fats are also less damaged by heat than monounsaturated fats found in olive oil, while the polyunsaturated vegetable fats found in shelf-stable oil products are damaged by harsh processing methods and undamaged polyunsaturated fats and oils should never be heated. Organic coconut products are therefore a healthy option for brain (and body) health.

WHICH SWEETENER IS BEST TO USE?

Most people have developed a sweet tooth due to the excessive amount of refined sugar that has insidiously found its way into our food supply. Using dates, maple syrup or coconut nectar to replace refined sugar in preparing treats is a first step towards improving choice of sweeteners; alternating with rice syrup (sometimes also called rice malt or brown rice syrup), which is very low in fructose, is a further improvement. Although honey has some health benefits, it is very sweet, and if consumed regularly it doesn't help reduce the desire for extremely sweet foods, which is the ultimate aim of a brain-friendly approach to eating. In addition, reducing the sweetness in these recipes is a great idea, as your sweet tooth becomes less demanding. Please keep in mind that using different sweeteners in baking can change the texture and look of baked goods.

WHICH PLANT-BASED MILK IS BEST TO USE IN SMOOTHIES AND DESSERTS?

Although there is now a large variety of plant-based alternatives to dairy milk, not all are created equal. Choose products that are sugar-free and organic. Although in these recipes I use a combination of plain coconut milk or an organic product that is made up of organic coconut and rice milk, to benefit from the nutrients that coconuts provide, you can use any plant-based milk. However, keep in mind that whichever plant-based milk you choose to use may influence the flavour of the dish. I use a mixture of coconut and rice milk in these recipes unless I mention the use of canned coconut milk or cream.

ARE FERMENTED FOODS GOOD FOR THE BRAIN?

Naturally fermented foods are good for the brain because they provide healthy probiotics — good bacteria — which help the digestive system work more efficiently. When the digestive system works well, both the quantity and the quality of the nutrients absorbed via the gut are optimized, which provides more nutrients for the busy brain (and body). There are many naturally fermented foods available today for purchase that you can easily add to your daily diet, and you can also make your own fermented foods, if you have the time and inclination.

GETTING STARTED

Although fresh is always better, some minimally processed foods are better than others, and can make preparing healthy food easier. Fresh fruit and vegetables should still be the backbone of 99 per cent of the food you prepare, but having the following basic foods on hand will help you make healthy meals and snacks quickly. (For processed food resources see page 228.)

STOCKING UP

Pantry

- ☐ Quinoa
- ☐ Millet
- ☐ Almond and/or peanut butter
- ☐ Tahini
- ☐ Brown basmati rice — uncooked and cooked
- ☐ Chickpeas (garbanzo beans) — uncooked and cooked in bottles/cans
- ☐ Lentils — uncooked and cooked in bottles/cans
- ☐ Artichokes
- ☐ Capers
- ☐ Tomato paste and pasta sauce in glass
- ☐ Dates
- ☐ Rice noodles
- ☐ Gluten-free pasta
- ☐ Coconut milk and cream
- ☐ A variety of spices
- ☐ Italian herbs
- ☐ Lemons
- ☐ Onions
- ☐ Garlic
- ☐ Sweet potato

Freezer

- ☐ Peas
- ☐ Sweet corn
- ☐ Frozen fruit, such as bananas and berries
- ☐ A variety of nuts and seeds

Please see www.lighterbrighteryou.life for Extra Resources — a brain-friendly shopping list

ACTIVATING NUTS

Soak nuts overnight in a glass bowl, with enough water to cover them (a ratio of 1:2, i.e. 1 cup of nuts for 2 cups of water), and rinse them well in the morning, under running water. They make great smoothies and snacks when they have been soaked and are left moist, although they have to be used up within about three days, and kept refrigerated to stop mould growing on them. I like to dehydrate them overnight, or for between 24 and 36 hours in the case of large nuts such as Brazils, in a 45-50°C/110-120°F oven, to bring back their crunch. They are then called 'activated' nuts, and consumers pay a premium when purchasing them because it is quite labour-intensive to make them. You can, however, make activated nuts quite easily in your own kitchen, as I do, making 2 kilograms (about 4½ pounds) at a time, storing them in the freezer and enjoying their extra nutrient density. They are super nutritious and very tasty either way.

COOKING LEGUMES

Although I prefer to use home-cooked legumes, having a few cans of legumes for emergencies is also a good idea. I look for companies that do not use bisphenol (BPA) as a lining in their cans— and only use tomato products in glass containers, because the acidity in tomatoes might react with any metal in cans. Always check the ingredients when purchasing canned foods: they only need to be in water, and salt is not necessary and preservatives are never needed. Cans used in my recipes are the standard size (420–440 grams/approximately 15 ounces.) A drained 425-gram can is the equivalent of 150 grams/5 ounces or 1⅓ cups cooked legumes (or ¾ cup of dried legumes). If there is another size, I will refer to it in precise terms. Dried legumes double their weight after being soaked, so when replacing them with canned legumes use half the weight of the canned legumes, i.e. for 250 grams (1 cup) of canned beans, use 125 grams (½ cup) dried beans. One cup of dried beans will produce approximately 1½ cups when cooked.

Red lentils and split peas do not require soaking, with red lentils cooking faster than split peas. Green lentils can go either way. Soaking will speed up cooking time, but if you've forgotten, you can easily cook them from scratch without it taking too much extra time.

Overnight soaking can also simply mean soaking the legumes while you are out during the day, with water added to them before you leave in the morning and having them ready to be drained and cooked when you get home late afternoon. Throw away the soaking water to get rid of the oligosaccharides (the sugars responsible for causing flatulence).

If you've forgotten to do the soaking, or don't have the time to do so, add three times the amount of water to the rinsed beans, bring them to the boil for a few minutes and then remove them from the heat, allowing them to sit for an hour. Discard the cooking water, then cook as per the recipe, or as if they had soaked overnight. This enables the seeds to absorb as much water in an hour as they would have absorbed in cold water overnight.

Generally speaking, the larger the seed, the longer the soaking time required, and the longer the seed soaks, the less time required for cooking. If you can easily crush the legume against the roof of your mouth with your tongue, it is cooked just right.

Follow the guide below, remembering that cooking times can vary depending on the age of the legumes. Do not add salt to legumes while they are cooking, because this can toughen them by reducing water absorption during cooking. Rather, add salt and other ingredients, such as tomatoes, which are acidic and can also stop cooking, after the beans are cooked. Do not add bicarbonate of soda (baking soda), because this decreases the vitamin B content of the beans. The amount of water you use will also influence the nutrient status of the end-product. Use twice the amount of water as lentils and split peas, and three times the amount for whole peas, beans and chickpeas (garbanzo beans). Adding more water than necessary will result in a loss of nutrients.

Cooking times for legumes after soaking

Adzuki beans	30–60 minutes
Black eye beans	1–½ hours
Borlotti (cranberry) beans	1 hour
Butter beans	1–1½ hours
Cannellini beans	1 hour
Chickpeas (garbanzo beans)	1½–2 hours
Flageolets	45 minutes
Haricot (navy) beans	1–1½ hours
Lentils — large brown/green	45 minutes
Mung beans	40 minutes
Red kidney beans	1–1½ hours
Soya (soy) beans	3–4 hours
Split peas — large	40–50 minutes

CONVERSION CHARTS

Oven temperatures

°Celsius (C)	°Fahrenheit (F)
120	250
150	300
180	355
200	400
220	450

Tip
I use a fan-forced oven, so if your oven does not use a fan you may have to increase baking time slightly.

Weight equivalents

Metric	Imperial (approx.)
10 g	⅓ oz
50 g	2 oz
80 g	3 oz
100 g	3½ oz
150 g	5 oz
175 g	6 oz
250 g	9 oz
375 g	13 oz
500 g	1 lb
750 g	1⅔ lb
1 kg	2 lb

Volume equivalents

Metric	Imperial (approx.)
20 ml	½ oz
60 ml	2 oz
80 ml	3 oz
125 ml	4½ oz
160 ml	5½ oz
180 ml	6 oz
250 ml	9 oz
375 ml	13 oz
500 ml	18 oz
750 ml	1½ pints
1 litre	1¾ pints

Cup and spoon conversions

1 teaspoon	5 ml
1 tablespoon	20 ml
⅓ cup	60 ml
¼ cup	80 ml
½ cup	125 ml
⅔ cup	160 ml
¾ cup	180 ml
1 cup	250 ml

The following chart is helpful when doubling recipes.

3 teaspoons	1 tablespoon
4 tablespoons	¼ cup
5⅓ tablespoons	⅓ cup
8 tablespoons	½ cup
10 tablespoons	⅔ cup
12 tablespoons	¾ cup
16 tablespoons	1 cup

USING BUCKWHEAT

Buckwheat is a nutrient-rich plant. It is a member of the rhubarb family, but due to the high quantity of edible seeds it produces it is mistaken for a carbohydrate grain (similar to quinoa) and therefore used as such. It is also a gluten-free food and is high in protein, containing all of the essential amino acids, as well as B vitamins, copper, iron, magnesium and manganese. So, it is not truly a carbohydrate, but it is used as one. Buckwheat is used to make soba noodles, which are a lovely way to enjoy a noodle-based salad (see page 103) without refined carbohydrates. It is great when soaked overnight in three times its amount of water, rinsed very well to get rid of the soapy residue, dried in a clean tea towel and then sprinkled with cinnamon and salt before being dehydrated in a preheated 40–45°C/105–110°F oven overnight until dry. Cool completely before storing in a glass container in the refrigerator and using as a topping on smoothies, sprinkled over salads and into cereals.

COOKING MILLET

Millet is a great gluten-free, nutrient-dense grain that easily replaces couscous or rice. Soaking millet overnight reduces its phytic acid content. Millet needs to be washed well in running water. Add 2¼ cups of water to 1 cup of millet and ¼ teaspoon salt to a saucepan and bring to the boil. Cover with a lid and reduce to a slow simmer for 25–30 minutes. Remove from the heat and set aside for about 10 minutes to allow the millet to complete cooking. Fluff lightly with a fork and serve immediately. Soaking the millet means you can use a ratio of 1:1½ (millet:water). By lightly roasting the grains before cooking, you enhance the nutty taste.

To bake millet, rinse it well and combine, in the ratio of 1 cup millet to 2½ cups water, in an ovenproof dish with a tight-fitting lid. Bake on 180°C/355°F for 30 minutes and then remove from the oven, leaving the lid on for about 10 minutes before serving. Keep in mind that 1 cup of uncooked millet yields about 3 cups of cooked millet.

COOKING QUINOA

Quinoa has a natural sticky coating called saponin, which is a bitter coating produced by the seed to keep insects from eating it before it has a chance to germinate. It is therefore best to rinse it before cooking to wash this bitter coating off the seed. (Some companies do this initial rinsing before packaging.) Soaking quinoa overnight will get rid of any saponin present and also reduce its phytic acid content. To cook quinoa, use this formula: 1 cup quinoa with 1½–2 cups water and ¼ teaspoon salt. If you want it very soft, use 2 cups of water, or use less for a little bite. Soaking quinoa for 8–10 hours (overnight) means that you can use a ratio of 1:1¼ (quinoa:water). Place the quinoa and water in a saucepan and simmer for 10 minutes. Remove the pan from the heat and let it sit covered for 5 minutes, or until all the liquid has been absorbed. Do not overcook — it will become mushy. It is light, fluffy and translucent and triples in quantity when cooked properly. Serve immediately. Its earthy flavour is great when served hot or cold. By lightly roasting the grains before cooking, you enhance the nutty taste. The uncooked grain should be stored in the refrigerator, because it spoils quickly.

A simpler method of cooking is to bring the quinoa and water to a rolling boil with the lid on, then turn the heat off and cover the lid snugly with a large, heavy dishcloth, and walk away. The residual heat will cook the quinoa in a few hours.

To bake quinoa, rinse it well and combine, in the ratio of 1 cup quinoa to 1¾ cups water, in an ovenproof dish with a tight-fitting lid. Bake on 180°C/355°F for 25 minutes and then remove from the oven, leaving the lid on for about 10 minutes before serving. Keep in mind that 1 cup of uncooked quinoa yields about 3 cups of cooked quinoa.

Note: Both quinoa and millet can be cooked in a rice cooker too, using the same water quantities and times.

NUT BUTTERS

Store-bought nut butters are not only more expensive than homemade ones, they may also contain sweeteners and be made using nuts that are past their prime and have been exposed to light and heat, making the nuts rancid with damaged fats, which are no good for your health. It's so simple to make your own using a combination of any nuts that appeals to you — once you get into the habit of doing so, you won't want to use anything else. Here are a few of the combinations that I use, and as long as you have a powerful blender, you won't need to add any other liquid (fat) to the mixture, because the nuts contain a lot of healthy fat that will naturally be released as the nuts break down and turn into a creamy butter. However, if you have a less powerful blender, you can still get a good result by adding a tablespoon or so of coconut oil, or even olive oil, to get the mixture moving. Feel free to experiment with your own mixtures. I use macadamia nuts in many of my combinations because they provide a subtle, natural sweetness to the butter. And you can also experiment with adding other ingredients to your nut butters — raw cacao powder, melted chocolate, vanilla essence or spices such as cinnamon and nutmeg. We enjoy adding some melted chocolate — a delicious treat on fresh, crispy apple slices!

NUT BUTTER (1)

1 cup macadamia nuts
1 cup cashew nuts

NUT BUTTER (2)

1 cup Brazil nuts
1 cup macadamia nuts

NUT BUTTER (3)

1 cup walnuts
1 cup cashew nuts

NUT BUTTER (4)

1 cup pecan nuts
1 cup macadamia nuts

Use these nut butters to stuff dates and dried apricots, spread onto apple and pear slices as a tasty snack and as a replacement for butter on toast and muffins.

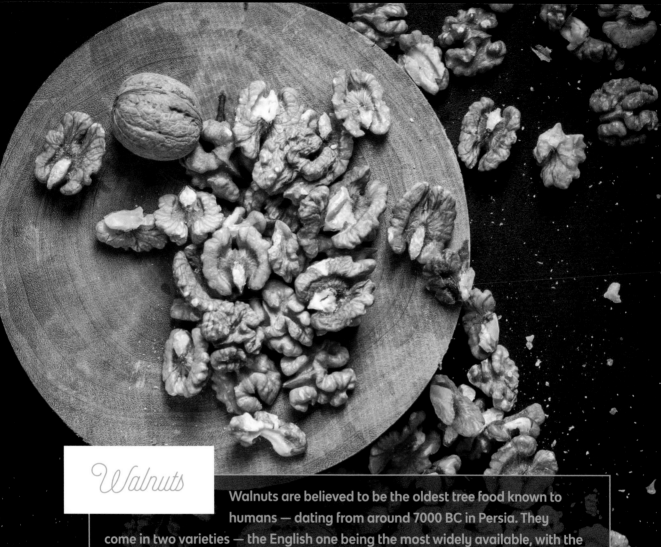

Walnuts

Walnuts are believed to be the oldest tree food known to humans — dating from around 7000 BC in Persia. They come in two varieties — the English one being the most widely available, with the familiar hard, tan shell; and the black walnut, with a stronger flavour. They are rich in the essential fatty acid (EFA) omega-6, although most people think they are full of omega-3s. In fact, they only have about 5 per cent omega-3, and 51 per cent omega-6, with the rest being made up of omega-9, which is what olive oil contains. EFAs, including omega-6, are critically important for brain health, and we have to get them from our diet — our body cannot make them! Walnuts also contain vitamin E, a potent fat-soluble antioxidant that the brain needs in great quantities. They also contain copper and manganese, as well as folic acid. There is even some evidence that they contain minute amounts of melatonin, which is great news for those who need some help in getting to sleep at night, because melatonin is the hormone produced in the brain when night falls and sleep beckons.

NUT CREAMS

Using cashew or macadamia nuts as the foundation, you can easily make a simple and delicious substitute for cream. I use this kind of cream over fruit salads, and over fresh berries as a delicious breakfast. The nuts are naturally sweet, so no added sweetener is needed. And, using the nuts to make a savoury cream is also a fabulous alternative to dairy cream, which is how we make gorgeous salad mayonnaises!

SWEET CREAM (MAKES 3 CUPS)

1 cup cashew or macadamia nuts, soaked for at least 4 hours or overnight, and drained

5–6 large ice cubes

1½ cups cold water

½ teaspoon vanilla essence

pinch of Himalayan salt

Blend all ingredients in a blender until smooth and creamy. Store the cream in an airtight glass container in the refrigerator for up to 5 days, where it will get thicker.

Variations

Replace the cashew nuts with macadamia nuts, which will result in a slightly sweeter cream.

Replace the water with coconut milk for a richer and creamier cream.

Add 1–2 pitted Medjool dates to slightly increase the sweetness.

To make a light pink cream, replace the ice cubes with 1 cup of frozen strawberries and process as per the original recipe, remembering that this cream will lose its vibrant pink colour quickly, so eat it all or store in the refrigerator and use within a day.

To make a savoury cream, use the same ingredients as above but add 1 large peeled garlic clove, the juice of 1 large lemon and ½ teaspoon herb salt. Add a little more lemon juice if you want to make a 'sour' cream, to use with the Mexican re-fried beans, for example (page 162). Using the nuts to make a savoury cream is also a fabulous alternative to dairy cream, which is how we make the gorgeous turmeric macadamia mayonnaise (see page 72).

GLUTEN-FREE FLOURS

Although there are many different kinds of gluten-free flours available in the store, I prefer to make my own, because then I know exactly what is in them. I use these two flours for different types of baking and make sure I always have a batch on hand to whip up some muffins or biscuits/cookies. (You can replace these homemade gluten-free flours with a store-bought gluten-free blend, but leave the baking powder out of the recipe if it's a self-raising blend.)

GLUTEN-FREE FLOUR (1)

2 cups chickpea flour (also called besan or gram flour)

1 cup brown rice flour

½ 1 cup potato starch*

½ 1 cup arrowroot or tapioca starch**

Combine these flours, then refrigerate in an airtight container and use as required.

Add 1 teaspoon baking powder per 1 cup flour for baking cakes and biscuits (cookies).

Note

* Potato starch and potato flour are made differently, and offer different qualities to baked goods. I prefer using potato starch in this mix, and suggest you do the same.

** Arrowroot and tapioca starch are different types of starch but can be used interchangeably — they are also sometimes called 'flours'.

GLUTEN-FREE FLOUR (2)

1 cup brown rice flour

1 cup arrowroot flour

½ cup quinoa flour

½ cup sorghum flour

Combine these flours, then refrigerate in an airtight container and use as required.

Use this combined flour in place of ordinary flour when baking biscuits/cookies (pages 218–22) or the spice and vanilla gluten-free cake (page 225).

Add 1 teaspoon baking powder per 1 cup flour for baking cakes and biscuits.

Blueberries

These smallish berries with a mild, sweet flavour are native to North America. Being extensively cultivated these days, they have become bigger, lacking the distinctive flavour of the wild fruit. Their deep blue pigment, a class of antioxidants called anthocyanins and proanthocyanidins, carries their powerful antioxidant ability, protecting the brain from the negative effects of ageing. These compounds also increase the levels of another important antioxidant called glutathione, which reduces brain inflammation and can play a major role in keeping the brain healthy. Research suggests that they can increase the ability of the brain to manufacture and release dopamine, and may also stimulate the pituitary gland to release growth hormone. This hormone is an anti-ageing hormone, and its synthesis slows down as we age.

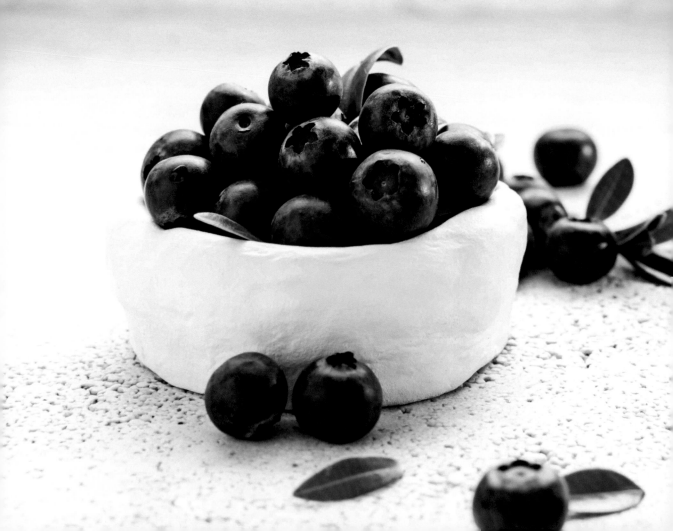

BREAKFASTS

Breakfast is a very important meal, especially for your brain. It has been managing overnight with stored forms of fuel and now requires a boost of nutrients to get you going and energized for a day filled with focused thinking and decision-making. The foods you choose to eat at this meal can set you up for a great day, or for cravings and unfocused thinking, as well as mood swings. Many cultures eat the same kinds of food for all their meals, so savoury breakfasts are nothing new, but they can be to westerners. When cereal became a favourite focus for breakfasts many decades ago, most people assumed that a sweet breakfast was the correct way to start the day. You may therefore be used to eating a sweet, cereal-based breakfast, but you will find healthier alternatives to store-bought cereals here. After all, starting your day with a very sweet breakfast can lead to blood-glucose swings that negatively affect brain function and mood. I've therefore also included some savoury breakfast ideas, many of which I enjoy regularly myself. Smoothies are many people's first choice for speedy breakfasts, but they need to be filled with the right kinds of nutrients, and have toppings to chew, otherwise they can lead to blood-glucose swings and cravings too. Remember to sit down and eat breakfast calmly and quietly, setting the scene consciously for a positive and productive day.

MAKE-YOUR-OWN GLUTEN-FREE GRANOLA

PREPARATION TIME: 30 MINUTES (PLUS OVERNIGHT BAKING TIME) | MAKES 4 CUPS

When you have a well-stocked pantry, refrigerator and freezer, it will be easy to make a batch of this crunchy and nutrient-dense cereal. The only thing you have to keep in mind is that it needs to 'bake' (dehydrate) overnight before you can eat it. You can use a variety of nuts, seeds and dried fruits (see the chart on page 38), and you can even adjust the kind of gluten-free flakes you use, for example, only using one of them, although I prefer to use the combination because then I'm increasing the nutrient density of this meal or snack. It's very crunchy, so soaking a few tablespoons in some of the melted ice-cream milkshake (see recipe on page 58) will soften it and increase nutrient density.

½ cup quinoa flakes

½ cup millet flakes

½ cup amaranth flakes

¾ cup rice, almond or coconut milk

½ cup coconut oil

½ teaspoon ground cinnamon

½ teaspoon mixed spice

½ teaspoon pure vanilla essence (vanilla extract)

¼ cup maple syrup, coconut nectar or rice syrup

⅓ cup cranberries

⅓ cup goji berries

5–6 dried apricots, finely chopped

½ cup almonds, roughly chopped

½ cup walnuts, roughly chopped

½ cup pecans, roughly chopped

½ cup Brazil nuts, roughly chopped

⅓ cup pumpkin seeds (pepitas)

⅓ cup sesame seeds

⅓ cup sunflower seeds

Preheat the oven to 50°C/120°F. Line a baking tray with baking paper. (You could also use a dehydrator.)

In a large bowl, combine the quinoa, millet and amaranth flakes. Mix well and set aside to allow the flakes to absorb the moisture, while you prepare the rest of the ingredients, which will take about 10 minutes.

Meanwhile, in a separate bowl, combine the remaining ingredients. Mix well so that they have a chance to stick together into smallish clumps with the oil, sweetener and spices.

Add the absorbed flakes to the oil mixture and combine well. Spread the mixture onto the baking tray — either break the mixture into smallish clusters to use as cereal or leave them larger as snacks — and 'bake' overnight (12 hours).

The next morning, check to see if the ingredients are all dry, and if not, stir them and continue dehydrating them for a few more hours.

When cool, store in an airtight glass container in the refrigerator for up to two weeks.

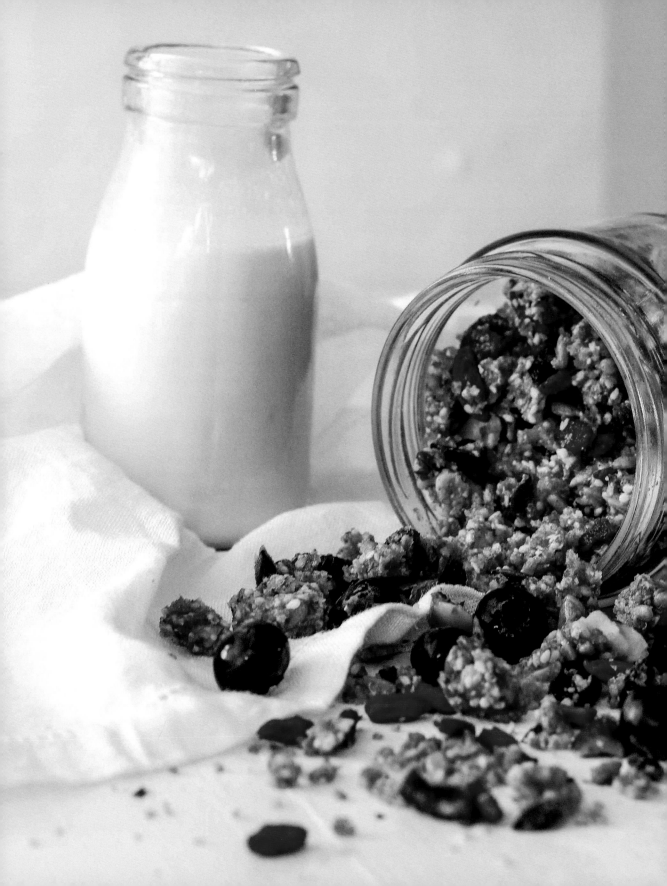

Make-your-own GF granola blueprint

Base (flakes)	Nuts	Seeds	Flavour	Sweet-ener	Liquid	Dried fruit	Topping
Quinoa	Almonds	Sesame	Vanilla	Rice syrup	Coconut oil	Apple	Coconut yoghurt
Amaranth	Brazils	Sunflower	Cinnamon	Maple syrup		Banana	Coconut milk
Millet	Cashews					Cherries	Rice milk
	Coconut	Pumpkin/pepita	Allspice			Cranberries	Almond milk
	Hazelnuts					Dates	Quinoa milk
	Macada-mias		Cacao			Goji berries	Fresh fruit — berries
	Pecans		Salt			Blueberries	
	Walnuts					Apricots	
						Mango	

Preheat the oven to 50°C/120°F. Line a baking tray with baking paper. You could also use a dehydrator.

Choose 1 cup of your base and add ½ cup nuts, ½ cup seeds and ½ cup dried fruit.

Heat ½ cup coconut oil and ¼ cup sweetener of your choice in a small pan over medium heat until just warm, adding the spices or flavouring of your choosing and a pinch of salt.

In a separate bowl, combine the dry ingredients and then mix with the oil mixture and bake overnight (12 hours).

When cool, store in an airtight glass container in the refrigerator for up to two weeks.

Variations
Add a few handfuls of puffed amaranth, millet or quinoa to the cereal when it has cooled to increase nutrients, texture and variety.

BREAKFAST GRANOLA BAR

PREPARATION TIME: 20 MINUTES | MAKES 24 SQUARES

When your time to have a leisurely, nutrient-dense breakfast runs out in the morning, it makes sense to have one or two of these bars handy. Not only are they simple to make, they are packed with brain-friendly nutrients and will keep you satisfied for many hours. The store-bought varieties are full of unnecessary sugars and damaged fats, so I much prefer to make my own. They are also great for preventing a mid-afternoon energy slump.

½ cup rolled quinoa flakes

1 cup roughly chopped pecans

1 cup roughly chopped almonds

¼ cup pumpkin seeds (pepitas)

¼ cup sesame seeds

¼ cup sunflower seeds

1 cup cranberries, roughly chopped

1 teaspoon pure vanilla essence (vanilla extract)

1 teaspoon ground cinnamon

¼ cup coconut nectar or maple syrup

¼ cup coconut oil

⅓ cup macadamia nut butter (see recipe on page 30)

In a large bowl, combine the quinoa, pecans, almonds, pumpkin seeds, sesame seeds, sunflower seeds and cranberries, and stir well.

In a large saucepan, combine the vanilla, cinnamon, sweetener and oil. Heat slowly over a medium heat, until bubbles form, then remove from the heat and stir in the macadamia nut butter.

Add the combined dry ingredients and mix well. Transfer the contents to a glass baking dish (9 x 5 centimetres/3½ x 2 inches) and press down hard, to flatten and smooth the top.

Using a sharp knife, cut into the mixture to make evenly sized squares or triangles, and refrigerate for a couple of hours until it is set.

Break into the pre-cut shapes and refrigerate in an airtight glass container for up to 10 days.

Variation
Replace the cranberries with dried blueberries, cherries or finely sliced dried apricots or dates.

Sunflower seeds

Sunflowers are a well-known symbol of summer, and their seeds were seen as a mystical symbol for the sun-worshipping Incas, who watched these beautiful flowers, with their seed-rich faces, follow its course through the sky. They contain a high percentage of omega-6 fats, as well as vitamins D, E and K, and some B vitamins. They also contain protein and pectin, a soluble form of fibre, so are a tiny but powerfully nutrient-dense brain food.

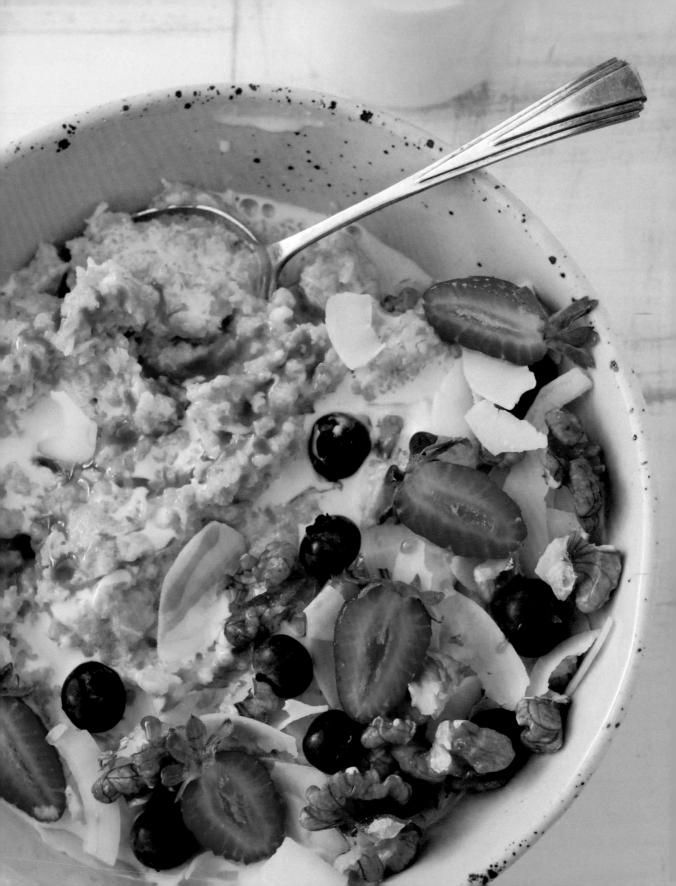

WARM GLUTEN-FREE BREAKFAST CEREAL

PREPARATION: 10 MINUTES | SERVES 4

If you want a warm, hearty breakfast on a cold day, try this recipe. Combine all the ingredients, choose a variation from the list below and you can quickly have a nourishing breakfast. When you keep on hand a variety of activated nuts, seeds and dried fruits you can make your own toppings with ease.

¼ cup quinoa flakes

¼ cup millet flakes

¼ cup amaranth flakes (or only one of these three)

2 cups coconut, rice or almond milk

2 tablespoons desiccated coconut

½ teaspoon pure vanilla essence (vanilla extract)

pinch of salt

In a large saucepan, combine all the ingredients and simmer over a medium heat for 15 minutes. Top with any of the variations below while the mixture is hot.

Variations

Sprinkle a handful of chopped almonds and blueberries over the top and then drizzle a drop of maple syrup or coconut nectar over the top.

Add a small handful of raspberries and a dollop of cashew nut cream and then top with a sprinkle of coconut sugar.

Sprinkle some cinnamon, nutmeg and all-spice over the top then add some grated apple and cranberries.

Sprinkle roughly chopped walnuts and pecans over the top and then add thinly sliced banana and dried cherries.

Tip

Cooked quinoa: Use ½ cup leftover quinoa (or that which you cooked on Sunday, see page 15) for breakfast, simply heating slightly with a little coconut, rice or almond milk, and add any of the variations above to make a satisfying breakfast.

Quinoa

Quinoa (keen-wah) is a high-protein food originating in South America that was a staple food of the Incas and Aztecs. It has been grown for 5000 years and has a long-standing reputation as a superb source of nourishment. It contains more protein than any other grain (50 per cent more than wheat) though it is actually a seed. It is very close to being a perfect food, being rich in vitamins and minerals, providing nearly four times more calcium than wheat, with more iron, phosphorous, lysine, zinc, manganese and magnesium, as well as vitamins A, E and Bs than other grains, all of which are important brain nutrients.

BANANA PANCAKES

PREPARATION TIME: 15 MINUTES | MAKES 12

These delicious pancakes can be thrown together in a few minutes. I do not like to fry food, but this recipe is an exception because you cannot have pancakes without frying being involved. I use coconut oil because it's not damaged by light, heat and oxygen exposure to the same extent that mono- and polyunsaturated fats are damaged.

1 cup almond flour

1 cup gluten-free flour 2 (see recipe on page 33)

½ heaped tablespoon psyllium husks

1 heaped teaspoon baking powder

pinch of salt

3 medium bananas, peeled and roughly mashed

1¼ cups water

½ teaspoon pure vanilla essence (vanilla extract)

coconut oil, for frying

cashew nut cream (see options on page 32), to serve

sliced bananas and strawberries, to serve

orange rind, to serve

maple or rice syrup, to serve

cinnamon, to serve

Preheat the oven to 50°C/120°F or its 'warm' setting.

In a large bowl, combine all the ingredients and mix well.

In a large non-stick frying pan, heat a few teaspoons of coconut oil over a medium heat. Spoon 2–3 ¼-cup measurements of the mixture into the pan (this will ensure that all the pancakes are the same size and cook uniformly) and fry for about 2 minutes on each side until the pancakes are slightly golden in colour, and then transfer to a warming plate in the oven. Continue this process until you've used up all the batter.

Serve the pancakes with cashew nut cream, sliced bananas and strawberries, orange rind and either maple or rice syrup and a sprinkle of cinnamon.

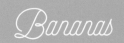

Bananas

The cultivation of bananas is believed to pre-date even that of rice. Technically a herb, bananas are the ultimate convenience food, coming in their own wrapping. They are best eaten when their flesh is marked with little brown spots, which indicates optimum ripeness. They contain significant amounts of potassium, manganese, vitamin B2 and vitamin B3, as well as fibre. Interestingly, they also contain a substance called fructooligosaccharide, or FCOS, which is a food for the probiotics (friendly bacteria) in your digestive tract and therefore called prebiotics. Our gut health is directly linked to our brain health, so apart from their nutrient content, they are a helpful 'gut-brain' food.

NUT AND SEED SNACK BAR

PREPARATION TIME: 10 MINUTES | MAKES 24 SLICES

You can eat this quick-to-prepare bar as a breakfast 'treat' or as a mid-afternoon snack. They are a little spicier than the breakfast granola bar (see page 39), and the addition of orange essential oil makes them more exotic.

2 cups desiccated coconut

½ cup walnuts

1 cup almonds

¼ cup pumpkin seeds (pepitas)

7 dates

½ cup dried apricots

½ cup dried cranberries

¾ cup tahini

3 tablespoons coconut oil

½ teaspoon ground cinnamon

½ teaspoon ground nutmeg

½ teaspoon dried ginger

4 drops organic essential sweet orange oil

¼ cup sesame seeds

Add the coconut to a food processor and mix until the coconut releases its oil, which will take 3-4 minutes.

Add the remaining ingredients, except for the sesame seeds, and pulse until all the ingredients are chopped well with only a few pieces of nuts and fruit left in small chunks.

Transfer the contents into a glass baking dish (9 x 5 centimetres/3½ x 2 inches) and sprinkle the sesame seeds over the mixture, pressing down firmly.

Using a sharp knife, cut the mixture to make evenly sized squares or triangles, and refrigerate for a couple of hours until it is set.

Break into the pre-cut shapes and refrigerate in an airtight glass container for up to 10 days.

Variations

If you have the time, roll the mixture into evenly sized balls and toss them in a mixture of coconut and raw cacao or carob powder.

Replace the tahini with cashew nut or macadamia nut butter.

Press a few tablespoons of puffed quinoa, amaranth or rice bubbles into the mixture before refrigerating.

GOLDEN POLENTA MUFFINS

PREPARATION TIME: 15 MINUTES | SERVES 12

These are our standard Sunday morning muffins. We vary the taste by adding either a cup of finely chopped dried figs, raisins and currants or, as a special treat, finely chopped dried Turkish apricots. If you use dried figs, simply add them to the rice milk to soften slightly while you're preparing the other ingredients. These muffins are quick to make, and when my children were younger they used to love doing the stirring, mashing and fruit chopping. We serve these muffins spread with a nut butter (see options on page 30).

coconut oil, to oil muffin tray

1 cup polenta

1 cup gluten-free flour 1
  (see recipe on page 33)

4 teaspoons baking powder

½ teaspoon psyllium husks

¼ teaspoon salt

1 teaspoon pure vanilla
  essence (vanilla extract)

2 ripe bananas, peeled and
  mashed

2 cups finely grated carrot

¼ cup coconut oil

1¼ cups rice or coconut milk

¼ cup maple or rice syrup

Preheat the oven to 190°C/375°F. Lightly oil a 12-hole muffin tray with coconut oil.

In a large bowl, combine the polenta, gluten-free flour, baking powder, psyllium and salt.

In a separate bowl, combine the vanilla, mashed banana, carrot, coconut oil, milk and syrup, then stir this mixture into the dry ingredients.

Spoon the mixture evenly into the muffin tray and bake for 12–15 minutes, until golden brown and firm to the touch. Remove the muffins from the oven and leave them to stand for about 10 minutes before removing them from the tray.

Variation
Replace the grated carrot with ½ cup each of roughly chopped pecans and dried cranberries.

Carrots

Carrots are actually part of the parsley family, so technically they are herbs. Carrot seeds have been found in ancient lake dwellings in Switzerland from 3000–2000 BC. They contain large amounts of vitamin A in the form of beta-carotene, as well as useful amounts of vitamins B3, C and E and the minerals calcium, potassium, iron and zinc, all important brain nutrients.

FOOD COLOURS

The pigments that colour the fruit (and vegetables) we eat are carried by powerful antioxidants!

Purple fruits contain flavonoids, including resveratrol, which help to keep our blood vessels healthy, improve immunity, may keep blood pressure stable and have been linked to vision and cognitive benefits. Choose raisins, red grapes, blackberries and mulberries.

Red fruits contain lycopene and vitamin C, powerful antioxidants that protect our digestive tract, stomach and lungs from cancer, as well as optimize immune function and healthy bones, teeth and skin. Choose watermelon, pink grapefruit, dragonfruit and pomegranates.

Yellow and orange fruits (as well as green kiwi fruit) contain carotenoids, such as beta-carotene, lutein and zeaxanthin as well as cryptoxanthin, which help to boost our immune system, feed our skin and act as potent antioxidants. Beta-carotene is converted into vitamin A, an important brain antioxidant. Choose bananas, mangoes, oranges, paw paws, passionfruit and kiwi fruit.

Green foods contain powerful antioxidants, such as glucosinolates and isothiocyanates, that contain cancer-fighting compounds, as well as lutein and zeaxanthin, potent eye nutrients. They also contain a vast array of other phytonutrients, many of which have as-yet undiscovered abilities to enhance our health and support our brain. Choose asparagus, broccoli, Brussel sprouts, kale, Chinese greens, rocket (arugula), watercress as well as seaweed produced from fresh, live plants.

Blue foods contain anthocyanins, along with lutein and zeaxanthin, which defend cells against cancer-forming compounds and prevent neuronal brain degeneration. Although researchers are not yet entirely sure why they are as powerful as they are, these compounds seem to be uniquely suited to quenching free-radical activity in the brain, even influencing neurotransmitter synthesis. Choose blueberries and dark cherries — blueberries contain more age-defying and disease-fighting antioxidants than any other vegetables or fruits.

Chia seeds

Chia seeds are part of the mint family and are native to Mexico, where the Aztecs used them as a main food as early as 3500 BC. They used these chia seeds for medicinal purposes, in drinks, and pressed them for oil, as well as during religious ceremonies. Today chia is grown in a number of Latin American countries but Australia is fast becoming a noteworthy producer. Chia seeds are tiny, nutrient-dense seeds that contain a number of important brain nutrients, such as the antioxidant vitamins A, C and E as well as a number of B vitamins. They are also high in calcium, magnesium and potassium and also contain iron and zinc. However, they are also high in omega-3, which makes them susceptible to damage if not refrigerated after harvesting. In addition, the omega-3 that they contain becomes more accessible when they have been soaked in liquid, because this softens their hard outer shell. Therefore, they are best soaked in water, or any of the options provided on page 16. Crushing them in a food processor after soaking makes their nutrients even more available. Due to their high omega-3 content it is best not to heat them in any way, because this causes damage to these delicate essential fats.

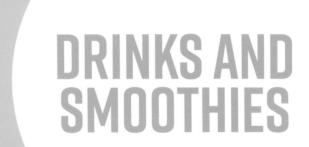

DRINKS AND SMOOTHIES

Optimal digestion and absorption, which starts with chewing food very well, is extremely important for optimal brain health. Most smoothies are just that, very smooth, and it's easy to just glug them down without thinking about the fact that they need to spend time in your mouth to stimulate digestive juices and also help your brain to register satiation. Crunchy, nutritious toppings added to smoothies therefore help you to slow down and focus on chewing the meal and enjoying the taste and texture. Here are my favourite toppings, but feel free to add what you love:

Buckwheat nibbles — soaked, drained and dehydrated buckwheat (see page 28)

Coconut 'chips' — strips of dried coconut

Activated nuts or seeds — any variety (see page 25)

Frozen or fresh berries — any variety

Handful of homemade granola (see recipe on page 36)

Two or three tablespoons of soaked chia seeds (see page 16)

MANGO, MACADAMIA AND COCONUT-MILK SMOOTHIE

PREPARATION: 5 MINUTES | SERVES 3

There is something seriously delicious and decadent about combining coconut milk, mango and macadamia nuts in a creamy smoothie — it tastes like dessert! Maybe it's because they are all tropical foods. Be sure to freeze peeled and sliced mangos when they are in season — you will so enjoy one of these smoothies when they are no longer readily available. One of our favourite ways to eat this smoothie is with fresh cherries.

2 cups mango pieces, either freshly sliced or frozen

⅓ cup macadamia nuts

1 cup coconut milk (or a combination of coconut milk and rice or almond milk)

½ cup coconut 'ice' cubes (see page 15)

pinch of turmeric

Combine all the ingredients in a blender and blend until smooth, thick and creamy. Serve topped with any of the choices on page 51.

Variation
Replace the macadamia nuts with any of your other favourites.

COLD CHOCOLATE AND COCONUT MILK

PREPARATION TIME: 5 MINUTES | SERVES 2

There are many store-bought coconut-and-chocolate drinks available, but reading the labels will reveal that most are filled with a variety of refined sugar, unnecessary additives and very few nutrients. My version, however, is delicious and can be whipped up in a few minutes if you have a blender. And the variations are endless. Enjoy! Remember to keep a stash of frozen coconut 'ice' cubes in your freezer (see page 15).

1 cup coconut milk

1 cup coconut 'ice' cubes (see page 15)

1 heaped tablespoon raw cacao powder

¼ cup macadamia nuts

3 large Medjool dates, pitted

¼ teaspoon pure vanilla essence (vanilla extract)

¼ teaspoon cinnamon

pinch of ground nutmeg

Combine all the ingredients in a blender and blend on high until smooth, thick and creamy. Serve topped with any of the choices on page 51.

Variations
Replace the macadamia nuts with cashew nuts.

To make a mocha drink, add ½ teaspoon instant decaffeinated powder (see resources on page 228 for an organic, healthy, decaffeinated instant coffee).

VERY BERRY AND CHERRY SMOOTHIE

PREPARATION TIME: 5 MINUTES | SERVES 2

Nothing beats a delicious homemade fruit smoothie — you know what's inside and you balance the flavours to suit yourself. This is a very nutrient-dense smoothie, and you can adjust it according to what berries you have on hand. Using only frozen berries ensures it stays cool and creamy even with a powerful blender.

2½ cups coconut milk

½ cup cashew nuts

1 cup cherries, pitted

1 cup blueberries

½ cup raspberries

1 teaspoon pure vanilla
   essence (vanilla extract)

Combine all the ingredients in a blender and blend until smooth, thick and creamy. Serve topped with any of the choices on page 51.

Variations

Replace the cashews with almonds or macadamias.

For a chocolate flavour, add 1 tablespoon of raw cacao powder.

Tip

Use the deep pink leftover water after boiling beetroots (beets) to soak some coconut flakes in and then dehydrate the flakes in a 60°C/140°F oven or dehydrator for a few hours until they are dry. You can sprinkle them over cakes or desserts for a nutritious visual and crunchy treat.

Cherries

Cherries are related to apricots, and therefore to the rose family, and are believed to be one of the oldest cultivated fruits. Due to their wonderful flavour they have graced the tables of emperors, conquerors and ordinary people. Their name originated from Latin, meaning 'for the birds', because birds love this fruit as much as we do. Cherries contain anthocyanins, potent brain antioxidants found in their deep reddish colour, as well as the eye nutrients lutein and zeaxanthin, and are helpful for inflammatory conditions. They also contain vitamins A and C, as well as calcium, magnesium and potassium. They are one of very few foods that contain melatonin, which is a natural hormone, produced in the brain, which helps to regulate sleep.

MELTED ICE-CREAM MILKSHAKE

PREPARATION: 5 MINUTES (PLUS OVERNIGHT TO SOAK THE ALMONDS) | SERVES 2

This is great as a dairy-free milk to pour over breakfast cereal. Add a banana for banana-flavoured milk, and replace the almonds with any other soaked nuts to enjoy a different flavour.

½ cup almonds, soaked in water overnight (about 10 hours)

4 Medjool dates, pitted

1 teaspoon pure vanilla essence (vanilla extract)

4 coconut milk 'ice' cubes (see page 15)

2 cups coconut milk

pinch of salt

Drain and rinse the almonds well (see page 25).

Combine all the ingredients in a blender and blend all together until smooth, thick and creamy. Serve as a milkshake or as milk over cereal.

Variations

Add ½ teaspoon each of cinnamon and nutmeg.

Add 1 tablespoon Teeccino dandelion caramel nut medium roast granules before blending (see resources, page 228).

MATTHEW'S 'YUM' DRINK

PREPARATION: 5 MINUTES | SERVES 4

My son designed this drink on a rainy, cold winter afternoon. He ensured everyone in the family enjoyed a mug and made me promise to include it in this book. If you don't enjoy carob, replace it with raw cacao, and if you don't have any rice milk use coconut milk instead. Adults might enjoy it with a drop of natural orange essential oil or some orange zest.

1 heaped tablespoon carob powder

3 cups rice milk

½ teaspoon pure vanilla essence (vanilla extract)

½ teaspoon cinnamon

4 large Medjool dates, pitted

½ cup cashew nuts

¼ cup almonds

pinch of salt

orange zest (optional)

Combine all the ingredients in a blender and blend until thick, warm and frothy. Serve with a sprinkle of carob or raw cacao powder.

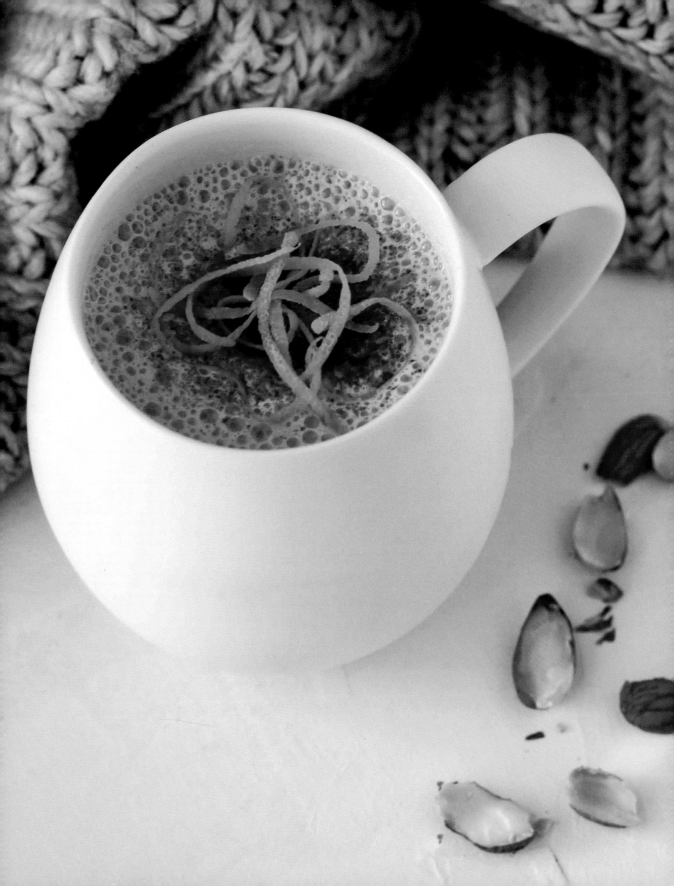

Olives and olive oil

Olives and olive oil are produced from one of the oldest and earliest cultivated trees in the world, being grown before written language was invented. Our best guess is that it was a native of Asia Minor and spread through Palestine, Syria and Iran to the Mediterranean region about 6000 years ago. When olive oil is produced from ripe, undamaged, healthy olives, which are processed within 24 hours of being picked, using simple, traditional, centuries-old methods, with no heat, and only mechanical pressing, the resultant oil is referred to as virgin olive oil. Olive oil contains 80 per cent monounsaturated fatty acids, 8–10 per cent omega-6 and about 1 per cent omega-3. The benefits of olive oil actually come from the minor ingredients that it contains, such as the following.

- Antioxidants, such as vitamin E, of which 88 per cent is in the form of alpha-tocopherol and beta-carotene (or pro-vitamin A), both with heart-protective properties.
- Magnesium-rich chlorophyll, which has many health benefits, including central nervous system (CNS) balance.
- Squalene, a precursor of phytosterols, which is heart protective via its antioxidant and cholesterol-balancing activities.
- Phytosterols, such as beta-sitosterol, which protect against cholesterol absorption.
- Modified sterols that have heart-health benefits.
- Polyphenols, which are responsible in part for the colour of olive oil, and have antioxidant capacities, including lowering blood pressure.
- More than 100 volatile compounds, which give olive oil its aroma and flavour, of which the benefits have not yet been discovered.

Remember to use only organic and cold pressed oils, as the damaged fats in refined oils are toxic to your delicate, fatty brain. Always keep olive oil in a dark cupboard rather than on the brightly lit countertop, because light causes oxidation of the delicate oil molecules. Never use any oils stored in plastic, because the chemicals in the plastic leach into the oil and you end up consuming them.

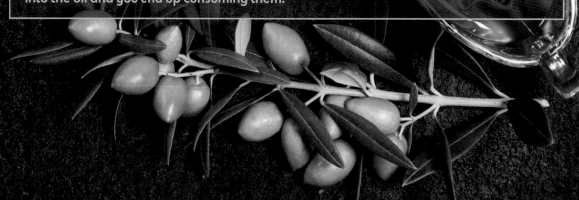

SAUCES, SALAD DRESSINGS, PESTOS AND SPICE BLENDS

A simple plate of vegetables, whether raw or cooked, wouldn't be particularly appetizing without some sort of condiment — even a splash of olive oil, a squeeze of lemon or lime juice and a sprinkle of sea salt can transform most vegetables into tastier morsels. Commercial salad dressings and sauces are filled with unpronounceable ingredients, which include preservatives, damaged fats, colourants and flavourings that do not add health to any salads.

I learned to make tasty dressings and sauces when my children were young, because I wanted to make sure that they would always associate eating vegetables with deliciousness. And because children love to dip their food into little bowls of sauces, I figured I would capitalize on this enjoyable activity.

These sauces, dressings and pestos, along with the spice blends, are all very adaptable and you can use them with any of the recipes in this book – and other foods that you prepare too. I prepare food by mixing and matching according to what I have on hand and what's in season, and this means that I stay flexible and creative. And you can easily do the same!

All the sauces, dressings and pestos will keep in an airtight glass container in the refrigerator for up to 5 days, although they never last that long in our home.

BASIC TOMATO SAUCE

PREPARATION: 5 MINUTES (PLUS 30–40 MINUTES COOKING TIME) | MAKES 5½ CUPS

A good tomato sauce is one of the cornerstones of any kitchen — here are three versatile sauces that you can use when tomato season is at its peak. However, I also keep a few bottles of a good organic tomato pasta sauce in my pantry for emergencies.

1 bottle (375 grams/13 ounces)
   tomato paste
   4 medium onions, peeled
   and roughly sliced

3½ cups water
   2 garlic cloves, peeled and
   chopped

3 tablespoons dried Italian
   herbs

2 tablespoons maple syrup

salt and pepper, to taste

¼ cup fresh basil, finely sliced

2 tablespoons olive oil

In a large saucepan, combine the tomato paste, onions, water, garlic, herbs, syrup and seasoning. Over a high heat, bring the mixture to the boil, then reduce to a simmer for 30 minutes or until the mixture has reduced to a thick sauce.

(Alternatively, you can place the tomato paste, onions, water, garlic, herbs, syrup and seasoning in a blender and blend briefly, then transfer to a saucepan and cook as required.)

Stir the basil leaves and olive oil into the sauce just before serving.

Any leftovers can be refrigerated in an airtight glass container and used within 5 days.

Variation

To transform this into pasta sauce, simply add a medium carrot (grated or roughly julienned) and a large capsicum (bell pepper) (seeded and sliced into strips).

Tip

A trip to the Seychelles taught me that certain spices, especially cinnamon, can enhance the flavour of a homemade tomato sauce immensely. Add 1½ teaspoons ground cinnamon, ½ tablespoon ground cumin, ½ tablespoon ground coriander and 2 tablespoons fresh ginger to the sauce as it starts cooking. It's great on roasted vegetables and on the pecan and bean burgers (see recipe on page 147).

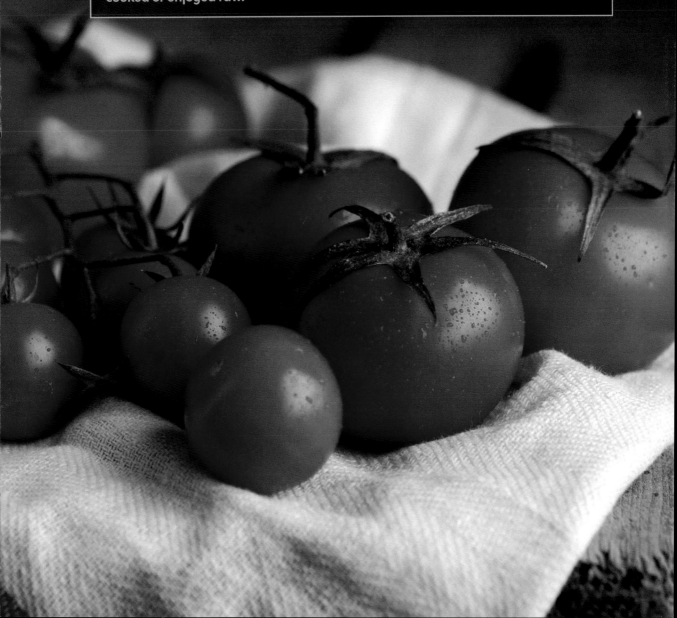

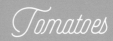

Tomatoes originated in the Andes area and were introduced throughout Europe and the western world around the 17th century. The early Italians named the tomato 'golden apple' and the French called them 'love apples'; they were thought to be an aphrodisiac. They contain vitamins C and E, as well as beta-carotene, magnesium, phosphorous and calcium. They also contain the bioflavonoid lycopene, which reduces the harmful effects of free radicals, which are released when our cells produce energy, and can be damaging to delicate brain cells The lycopene they contain is effective whether tomatoes are cooked or enjoyed raw.

ROASTED TOMATO SAUCE

PREPARATION: 2½ HOURS | MAKES 2–3 CUPS

When there is a glut of tomatoes at the markets at the height of summer I make a batch of this special, rich sauce. Use it as a quick pasta sauce, on gluten-free pizzas or simply as a pesto-like spread for crackers. This is summer flavour at its best; the tomatoes break down into a luscious blend of gorgeous flavour, and the garlic and herbs add extra depth.

1 kilogram (2¼ pounds) fresh, ripe tomatoes

10 garlic cloves, peeled and sliced

1 cup fresh basil, finely sliced

salt and pepper, to taste

Preheat the oven to 100°C/210°F. Line a baking tray with baking paper.

Soak the tomatoes in boiling water for a few minutes, then slip their skins off and remove their stem. Cut the tomatoes into thick slices, then lay them on the baking tray and bake for 1 hour.

Remove from the oven and insert the garlic slices into the tomato slices. Cover them with a sheet of baking paper so that they don't burn, and return the tray to the oven. Bake for a further hour, until the juices seep out of the tomato slices, and the garlic has baked through.

Remove from the oven and pour the mixture into a large bowl, adding the basil and seasoning with salt and pepper.

Allow the mixture to cool and then store in an airtight glass container in the refrigerator, with a layer of olive oil spread over the top. Use as a pasta sauce, a soft pesto or cracker spread. Any leftovers can be refrigerated in an airtight glass container and used within 5 days.

Variations

If you can also find luscious red capsicums (bell peppers), simply grill two or three (see page 71), then peel, slice thinly, and add to the finished sauce.

For a smoother sauce, blend briefly in a food processor.

PAPRIKA-SPICE SAUCE FOR GRILLED VEGETABLES

PREPARATION: 15–20 MINUTES | MAKES 2 CUPS

This is a rich, tasty sauce to serve with grilled vegetables and quinoa. It has a lovely spicy flavour, but no heat, so if you'd like some heat add a teaspoon or so, according to your taste, of freshly sliced chilli (chili pepper).

1 can (400 millilitres/12 fluid ounces) coconut cream

2 large garlic cloves

1 tablespoon fresh ginger, finely chopped or 2 teaspoons ground, dried ginger

½ medium onion, peeled

3 teaspoons cumin seeds

2 teaspoons sweet Hungarian paprika

¼ teaspoon cardamom seeds, out of the pod

juice of 1 large lime or 1 medium lemon

1 large pinch sea salt flakes

2 kaffir lime leaves, spine removed

bunch of fresh coriander (cilantro), separated into 2 halves, one half finely sliced and set aside

Combine all the ingredients except for the coriander in a blender. Blend on high until well combined and all the seeds are finely crushed.

Add the unchopped half of the coriander and pulse briefly, then pour the mixture into a saucepan. Place over a medium heat for 10 minutes to reduce slightly before serving.

Add the remaining sliced coriander just before pouring over roasted vegetables. Any leftovers can be refrigerated in an airtight, glass container and used within 5 days.

MANGO MUSTARD SALAD DRESSING

PREPARATION: 5 MINUTES | MAKES 1½ CUPS

When mango season arrives we make this dressing a lot. It's very fresh and light and the colour is gorgeous — and it contains loads of great nutrients too. This dressing is delicious served on a combination of rocket (arugula) and baby spinach leaves with slivers of artichoke hearts, marinated onion (see page 16) and avocado.

1 cup mango, sliced from fresh or frozen

¼ cup olive oil

juice of 1 medium lemon or 2 small limes

½ teaspoon herb salt

1 teaspoon mustard powder

2 tablespoons water

Combine all the ingredients in a food processor and blend until thick and creamy. Serve with a crispy green leaf salad.

Refrigerate in an airtight glass container for up to 5 days.

Variation
Replace the olive oil with coconut cream for a creamier version.

TAHINI HERB SALAD DRESSING

PREPARATION: 10 MINUTES | MAKES 2 CUPS

Use this dressing for lightly steamed vegetables, as a raw salad dressing or as a dip for fresh, raw vegetables. Even those people who find the taste of tahini rather exotic and strange at first, enjoy this dressing. It is packed full of easily absorbable calcium — so children will benefit from dipping their fresh vegetable sticks into this mixture. As tahini is a natural product and the texture can vary, if it seems too thick just add some more water and blend a little more.

1 cup tahini

1 cup water

juice of ½ a lemon

1 large garlic clove, peeled

½ teaspoon herb salt

1 teaspoon paprika

1 large spring onion (shallot, scallion), roughly chopped

1 teaspoon fresh basil, finely chopped

1 teaspoon fresh oregano, finely chopped

Combine the tahini, water, lemon juice, garlic, herb salt, paprika and spring onion in a blender and blend until light and creamy. Stir in the basil and oregano, or add to the blender and pulse briefly.

Refrigerate in an airtight glass container for up to 5 days.

Variation
Replace the fresh herbs with ½ teaspoon dried Italian herbs.

TOMATO SALAD CREAM DRESSING

PREPARATION: 10 MINUTES | MAKES 2 CUPS

Children of all ages enjoy dipping their crunchy vegetables or oven-baked sweet potato chips into this salad cream — and it is much healthier than store-bought sauces. It is good with all fresh vegetable salads as well as grain salads but looks especially appealing on green salads, because the pink contrasts beautifully with green leaves.

1 small (10-centimetre/ 4-inch) piece celery, roughly chopped

1 spring onion (shallot, scallion) , roughly chopped

¼ cup tomato paste

3 tablespoons lemon juice

1 large garlic clove, peeled

½ teaspoon herb salt

¾ cup coconut milk

Combine all the ingredients in a blender and blend until smooth and creamy. Serve as a dipping sauce or with the gorgeous green garden salad on page 96.

Refrigerate in an airtight glass container for up to 5 days.

RASPBERRY SALAD DRESSING

PREPARATION: 5 MINUTES | MAKES 1½ CUPS

Raspberries are gorgeous in colour and have a distinct flavour as well as a large supply of antioxidants and fibre. This dressing is very simple to make with either fresh or frozen raspberries, and delivers a tasty hit of flavour to any salad with green leaves. It's one of our favourites!

1 cup raspberries (frozen or fresh)

2 tablespoons maple syrup

¼ cup olive oil

¼ cup lemon juice

¼ teaspoon herb salt

Combine all the ingredients in a glass bowl. (If you are using frozen raspberries, allow them to thaw.)

Lightly crush the berries with a fork so that the whole mixture turns light pink, then transfer the mixture to a small pouring jug and stir well before each serve.

Refrigerate in an airtight glass container for up to 5 days.

Variation
Replace the raspberries with chopped blueberries.

INSTANT MAYONNAISE

PREPARATION: 5 MINUTES | MAKES 1½ CUPS

This is the quickest mayonnaise you'll ever make! It can be used in stuffed sweet potatoes, as a dip for crisp raw vegetables, over any salad or spread on crackers. It's especially good with fresh asparagus. You can whip it up in a few minutes when you have an emergency dressing to make. Snip a few herbs into the mixture after blending and you have a colourful and tasty alternative to shop-bought mayonnaise. Enjoy!

1 bottle (425 grams/15 ounces) artichokes, drained

½ cup olive oil

¼ cup water

1 garlic clove, peeled

1 teaspoon herb salt

¼ teaspoon ground cumin

2 tablespoons fresh lemon juice

Combine all the ingredients in a blender and blend until thick and creamy.

Refrigerate in an airtight glass container for up to 5 days.

Artichokes

Artichokes are native to Europe and North Africa. They contain silymarin, a flavonoid that helps protects liver cells and cell membranes, by aiding liver detoxification; and also cynarin, an antioxidant that helps the liver produce bile, which is the substance that helps the liver process fat, as well as helping the flushing of toxins from the cells. Both of these compounds also help to regenerate liver cells. They contain vitamins A and C, as well as calcium, potassium, iron and fibre. They also contain a huge amount of fibre, up to 10 grams per artichoke heart, so help the bowel detoxify naturally too, and they provide nourishment for our good bowel bacteria, so are also known as prebiotics. A healthy liver and gut help the brain to work more efficiently.

CORIANDER (CILANTRO) AND PINE NUT MAYONNAISE

PREPARATION: 10 MINUTES | MAKES 1½ CUPS

Any salad becomes inspired with a drizzle of this pale green mayonnaise. The pine nuts lend a rich flavour, while the ginger gives this dressing plenty of zing. You can also sprinkle some soya (soy) sauce over the salad after dressing it with this mayonnaise — the ginger, coriander (cilantro) and soya sauce work together superbly. The Chinese greens and baked tofu salad on page 116 goes well with this dressing. Use it instead of ordinary mayonnaise for a tasty change.

¼ cup olive oil

½ cup pine nuts

1 cup chopped fresh coriander (cilantro)

2 teaspoons grated fresh ginger

2 tablespoons lemon juice

6 tablespoons water

1 small garlic clove, peeled

salt and pepper, to taste

Combine all the ingredients in a blender and blend until thick and creamy — as it stands it will get thicker.

Refrigerate in an airtight glass container for up to 5 days.

Variation
Replace the pine nuts with cashew nuts.

QUICK GARLIC AND MUSTARD DRESSING

PREPARATION: 10 MINUTES | MAKES ¾ CUP

This is a quick dressing that doesn't require the use of a food processor. Simply make it in a small bowl, throw it over your salad, toss and eat immediately. It is good with any of the leafy salads in this book (see pages 89–117) and is lovely over a simple salad of sliced tomato and avocado.

2 garlic cloves, crushed or finely chopped

½ cup olive oil

juice of 1 medium lemon

1 tablespoon maple or rice syrup

1 teaspoon mustard powder

salt and pepper, to taste

In a bowl, combine all the ingredients and stir until smooth. (Alternatively blend in a blender.) Pour over salad, toss, and serve immediately.

Refrigerate in an airtight glass container for up to 5 days.

ROASTED GARLIC DRESSING (I)

PREPARATION: 10 MINUTES (PLUS 40 MINUTES TO ROAST THE GARLIC) | MAKES 1 CUP

Roasted garlic is a wonderful ingredient — the roasting process gives this bulb a buttery flavour and a creamy texture that can enhance most vegetable dishes. This simple dressing is great over most salads, and pouring this over baby steamed beetroots (beets) is a match made in culinary heaven!

2 tablespoons fresh lemon juice

1 teaspoon maple or rice syrup, or coconut nectar

½ teaspoon dry mustard

5 large roasted garlic cloves, peeled (see tip)

½ cup olive oil

pinch of turmeric

salt and pepper, to taste

Combine all the ingredients in a blender and blend until smooth.

Refrigerate in an airtight glass container for up to 5 days.

Variation

Add fresh herbs to this mixture for a change of taste, such as fresh basil, fennel, coriander (cilantro), lemon thyme or oregano.

Tip

Roasting garlic brings out the rich, mellow flavour of garlic, without the bite. Preheat the oven to 160°C/320°F. Wrap the whole bulb in baking paper and place on a baking tray. Bake for about 40 minutes, then allow to cool. Either separate the cloves to use separately, or use as a spread by squeezing all the garlic out of the cloves and adding to a blender or food processor with ¼ cup olive oil and a pinch of salt, or mash all with a fork. The resultant white cream can be spread onto fresh bread, added to pâtés, soups, used as a butter in baked sweet potatoes and with roasted vegetables to impart a warm, mellow garlic flavour. Roasted (peeled) garlic cloves are also a great ingredient in salad dressings.

CANNELLINI AND ALMOND 'HUMMUS'

PREPARATION: 10 MINUTES | MAKES 1½ CUPS

Traditional hummus is made with cooked chickpeas (garbanzo beans) and tahini, but here we shake it up a little by substituting cannellini beans and almonds for the chickpeas, thereby increasing the nutrient density and losing none of the flavour — or usefulness.

1⅓ cups cooked cannellini beans (or 425 gram/15 ounce can), drained

1 large garlic clove, peeled

⅓ cup almonds

3 tablespoons tahini paste

juice of 1 lemon

½ teaspoon ground and roasted cumin

½ teaspoon ground coriander

1 teaspoon smoked paprika

salt and pepper, to taste

olive oil, to sprinkle

Combine the cannellini beans, garlic, almonds, tahini, lemon juice, cumin, coriander and paprika in a food processor and blend until smooth and creamy. Taste and season with salt and pepper. Sprinkle olive oil over the top to serve.

Refrigerate in an airtight glass container for up to 5 days.

Variations

After processing, add 1 cup of roughly chopped fresh coriander (cilantro) and pulse briefly.

To make red capsicum (bell pepper) hummus, add a grilled, cooled, peeled and de-seeded red capsicum (see page 71) before processing.

MUSHROOM PÂTÉ

PREPARATION: 30 MINUTES (PLUS 2–3 HOURS TO SOAK THE PORCINI) | MAKES 1½ CUPS

When I found this recipe, the photograph looked so good that I wanted to make it immediately. However, it was full of butter, cream and port, so I decided to adapt it. The result is every bit as delicious, only healthier.

1 cup (25–30 grams/1 ounce) dried porcini mushrooms

1 cup water

1 small onion, peeled and finely chopped

1 garlic clove, crushed

2 cups chopped fresh mushrooms such as button and big brown

salt and pepper, to taste

¼ teaspoon freshly grated nutmeg (optional)

½ cup cashew nut cream (see options on page 32)

1 tablespoon lemon juice

After washing the porcini very well under running water to get rid of any small pieces of sand or twigs, place them in a bowl with 1 cup of water. Allow them to soak for 2–3 hours, then strain through a very fine sieve (or clean coffee filter) to catch any sand or twigs, and set the water aside. Wash the porcini well again under running water and transfer the porcini to a saucepan.

Add the onions, garlic, mushrooms and ⅓ cup of the strained soaking water to the saucepan and cook (with lid on) over medium heat for about 20 minutes, or until the mushrooms are cooked and most of the moisture absorbed. Remove from the heat and set aside to cool.

Season with salt and pepper, and add the nutmeg if using. Transfer the mixture to a food processor and blend briefly so as to retain a few chunks.

Remove from the food processor. Add the nut cream and lemon juice, stirring well, then refrigerate in an airtight, glass container for 2 hours. Serve with crisp vegetable sticks or on rice or quinoa crackers.

Refrigerate in an airtight glass container for up to 5 days.

Variation
If the flavour of nutmeg doesn't appeal to you, use lemon thyme instead. Simply chop about 2 tablespoons finely and sprinkle that into the mixture before you refrigerate it.

GRILLED EGGPLANT (AUBERGINE) PÂTÉ

PREPARATION: 40 MINUTES | MAKES 3 CUPS

We invented this pâté when we had too many eggplants — and we added coriander (cilantro) because it's my daughter's favourite herb. The addition of roasted garlic was due to us having discovered what a wonderfully creamy and subtle flavour roasting gives this versatile bulb. The result is a delicious pâté, which is equally good with fresh vegetables, on a gluten-free cracker or as a filling for a baked potato. Only add the olive oil if the mixture is too thick — generally the juices from the eggplant ensure a thin-ish mixture.

2 large or 3 medium eggplants (aubergine)

3 garlic cloves, peeled and roasted (see page 70)

2 tablespoons olive oil (optional)

3 tablespoons tahini

juice of 1 large or 2 small lemons

1 small onion or 3 spring onions (shallots, scallions), peeled and finely chopped

salt and pepper, to taste

½ cup fresh coriander (cilantro), roughly chopped (optional)

Preheat the oven to 180°C/355°F. Line a baking tray with baking paper.

Cut the stem from each eggplant and lay the eggplants on the tray. If you don't have any roasted garlic, simply roast the cloves, wrapped in baking paper, at the same time. Roast the eggplant (and garlic) for about 30 minutes or until the skin is blackened. Remove from the oven and transfer the eggplant (and garlic) to a bowl, cover and set aside to cool.

Peel the eggplants (and garlic) and add the pulp to a food processor, along with the remaining ingredients. Mix quickly, allowing the mixture to remain somewhat chunky.

Refrigerate in an airtight glass container for up to 5 days.

Tip

Simply put your fresh eggplant on a grill, turning regularly until the skin is blackened and the vegetable becomes soft. Transfer to a large glass bowl and cover with a tea towel. When they are cool enough to handle, remove the black skin and you are left with lovely cooked flesh. You may have to drain the flesh to get rid of some of the juices. If you don't have a grill, simply put the eggplants into a hot oven (190°C/375°F), with the grill on, for about 30 minutes, turning regularly until the skin is blackened, and continue as above.

PEANUT SATAY SAUCE

PREPARATION: 10 MINUTES | MAKES 1½ CUPS

This quick-to-make sauce is very useful when you've made a stir-fry and want a tasty topping. It beats the store-bought varieties hands down and is naturally a lot healthier. It doesn't matter whether the peanut butter is chunky or smooth. Serve with the noodle salad on page 103, and with the kale stir-fry on page 169.

6 tablespoons peanut butter
1 large garlic clove
juice of ½ large lemon
1 cup coconut milk
½ teaspoon salt

Combine all the ingredients in a blender and blend until creamy, smooth and slightly warm. Pour the mixture into a jug to serve.

It can be used the next day too, cold from the fridge, as a dip for lightly steamed broccoli or cauliflower.

Refrigerate in an airtight glass container for up to 5 days.

Variation
Add a pinch of dried ginger or ½ teaspoon grated fresh ginger.

Garlic

Garlic is the most famous member of the onion family and has more superstition and folklore surrounding it than any other food. Pyramid-building slaves are believed to have refused to work unless they were given garlic to eat, believing it gave them great strength. In Shakespeare's time it was regarded as an aphrodisiac (presumably if both parties partook of it!). Egyptian papyri list 22 prescriptions using garlic, while vampires are supposedly repelled by it. The flavour is milder when it is sliced or used whole, whereas crushing it releases a stronger flavour. Garlic contains powerful natural antibiotics, along with antifungal and antiseptic properties. It's a natural blood-thinner and cholesterol-lowering food, and contains vitamin B6, iron, phosphorous, potassium, manganese and selenium as well as allicin, a health-promoting sulphur compound. Eating parsley, mint or fennel seeds will help to get rid of 'garlic breath'.

NIGHTSHADE SAUCE

PREPARATION: 45 MINUTES | MAKES 2 CUPS

Eggplants (aubergine), capsicums (bell peppers) and tomatoes (as well as white potatoes) belong to the nightshade family of vegetables. This is a summer dish, which can be made with great ease when this produce is plentiful. It also smells wonderful while it's baking, and is versatile — you can use it as a pasta sauce (double or triple the quantities, because you would need about ½ cup of this sauce per bowl of pasta) or as a topping for a green salad, as a great dip for spicy sweet potato 'chips' (see recipe on page 175) or even as a topping for burgers (see recipe on page 147).

1 medium eggplant
  (aubergine)

1 red capsicum (bell pepper)

4–5 ripe tomatoes

7–8 large garlic cloves

sprinkle of herb salt

¾ cup loosely packed fresh
  basil leaves

salt and pepper, to taste

Preheat the oven to 180°C/355°F. Line a baking tray with baking paper.

Cut the eggplant in half and lay it cut face down on the tray.

Cut the capsicum in half, remove the seeds and lay it cut face down on the tray.

Cut the tomatoes in half and lay them cut face down on the tray.

Twist the garlic cloves into a strip of baking paper and lay on the tray with the rest of the vegetables.

Sprinkle with a little herb salt and bake for 30–40 minutes or until the vegetables are cooked and the skin of the capsicum and tomatoes has blistered.

Remove from the oven and allow the vegetables to return to room temperature before you scoop the flesh out of the eggplant, and remove the skin from the capsicum (pepper) and tomatoes.

Chop the flesh of the vegetables roughly, then toss with the basil and olive oil and serve at room temperature with spicy sweet potato 'chips', tossed into a pasta or over a green salad.

Store in the refrigerator in an airtight glass container for up to 5 days.

Variation
If you don't have any fresh ripe tomatoes on hand, soak 1 cup sun-dried tomatoes in water for about an hour and then squeeze them dry.

SPICY HARISSA SAUCE

PREPARATION: 15 MINUTES | MAKES 1½ CUPS

This sauce is a spicy, hot blend of ingredients that have been combined and used in Tunisian cooking for hundreds of years — although it has been called a Moroccan sauce. It adds heat to anything — I've known people to add this mixture to salads, spread it on gluten-free crackers and even put it into baked sweet potatoes and as a topping for pecan and bean burgers (see recipe on page 147). Use it wherever you want a hit of flavour.

2 tablespoons ground coriander

2 tablespoons ground cumin

2 tablespoons crushed dried red capsicum (crushed red pepper)

1 tablespoon black pepper

3 garlic cloves

2 medium (1 cup) Jalapeño peppers, seeded

2 medium red capsicums (bell peppers), roasted (see page 71)

juice and rind of 1 small lemon or lime

¼ cup olive oil

salt, to taste

Combine all the ingredients in a blender and blend until smooth and creamy.

Refrigerate in an airtight glass container for up to 2 weeks, covered with a layer of olive oil.

Variation
Replace the raw garlic cloves with 1 head of garlic, peeled and roasted (see page 70).

AVOCADO SALSA

PREPARATION 15 MINUTES | MAKES ABOUT 5 CUPS

A salsa is a combination of a salad and a sauce. Use it to smother the pecan and bean burgers on page 147 or to top the re-fried beans on page 162. Sometimes it's nice to just eat it alone with some baked corn 'chips'. Leaving out the ground spices will result in a more traditional avocado guacamole dish.

2 large avocados

1 small lemon or lime

1 small red capsicum (bell pepper), finely chopped

1 medium tomato, cut into small cubes

1 teaspoon ground cumin

1 teaspoon ground coriander

1 medium red onion, peeled and finely chopped

1/3 cup chopped fresh coriander (cilantro)

3-4 tablespoons olive oil

a few chilli (chili pepper) flakes (optional)

salt and pepper, to taste

Peel and chop the avocados into medium-sized cubes and place in a large bowl. Add the juice from the lemon or lime and then the remaining ingredients, mixing carefully so as to retain some of the avocado cubes (do not mash them all).

(If you are in a hurry, simply combine all the ingredients in a food processor and pulse the mixture a few times. You will end up with some smallish pieces and some larger ones.)

Refrigerate in an airtight glass container until needed — only for a few hours — and let the mixture return to room temperature before serving. (Avocados do not lend themselves to overnight refrigeration, so it's best to eat this on the day that you make it.)

Avocados

Avocados are members of the bay tree family. The first known record of the avocado is in Mayan and Aztec picture-writings from 3000 BC. They are picked when mature — but not ripe. They contain vitamins A, B1, B2, B3, B5, B6, vitamins C and E as well as folate, iron, magnesium, potassium and mostly omega-9 monounsaturated fats. Avocados are truly one of nature's wonder foods, containing many brain nutrients.

SALSA VERDE

PREPARATION: 15 MINUTES | MAKES ABOUT 1½ CUPS

This is a lovely green sauce, which is packed with nutrients and can be used in a variety of wonderful ways to add something special to your ordinary, day-to-day meals. It will lose its lovely green colour very quickly, so cover it with a layer of oil before storing in the fridge — or even better, use it shortly after making it. You can use this sauce over roasted vegetables, as a dip for fresh veggies or as a chunky salad dressing. It's also great served over buckwheat noodles for a fresh cold noodle salad or even as the final topping for stuffed sweet potatoes.

1 cup flat-leaf parsley

½ cup mint leaves

½ cup basil leaves or dill leaves

1 large garlic clove

2 tablespoons salted capers, soaked and rinsed well to get rid of most of the salt

2–3 tablespoons lemon or lime juice

¼ cup olive oil

pepper, to taste

Combine all the ingredients in a food processor and pulse in quick bursts, to leave the mixture chunky.

Use immediately or refrigerate in an airtight glass container for up to 5 days, covered with a thin layer of olive oil.

Variation
Replace the basil and parsley with coriander (cilantro) leaves, and add a few kaffir lime leaves (their spine removed).

Parsley

Parsley is one of the oldest known herbs, and its history is shrouded in the mists of time. This herb is full of vitamin A in the form of beta-carotene, vitamin C, as well as vitamins E and K, folate, calcium, iron, magnesium potassium, manganese, zinc, phosphorous and copper. Parsley is also full of lutein and zeaxanthin, promoting good eye health, along with other brain antioxidant benefits

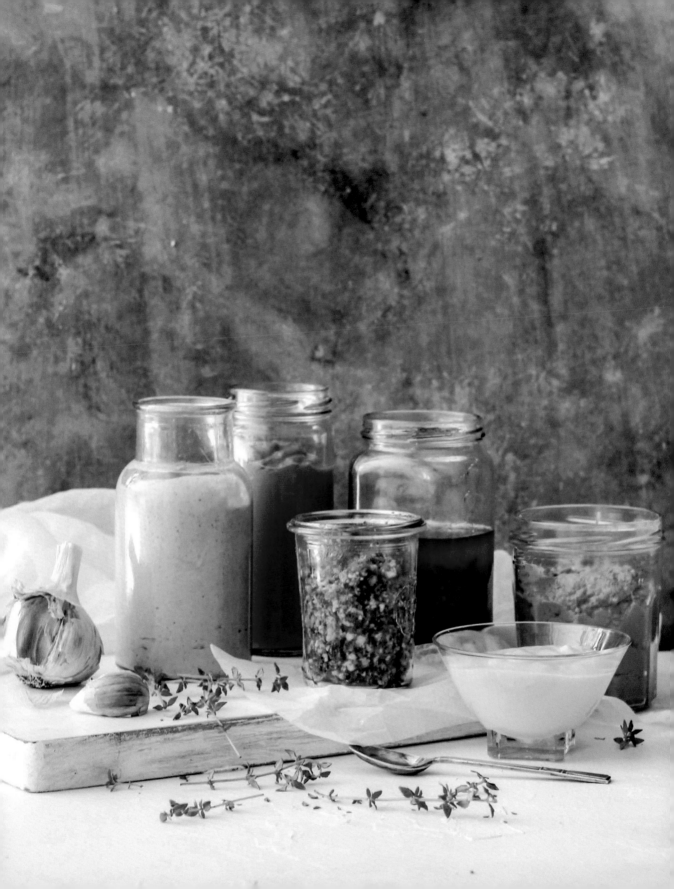

HERB AND CAPSICUM (BELL PEPPER) OILS

PREPARATION: 5 MINUTES | MAKES 1½–2 CUPS

Herb oils can be used in a variety of ways — over salads as a basic, refreshing dressing; over roasted vegetables; and over rice or quinoa pilafs. They add flavour and nutrients — and of course, visual appeal.

Coriander (cilantro) oil

We pour this oil over salads, onto oven-baked sweet potato 'chips' (see recipe on page 175) and over vegetable and grain pilafs such as the currried carrot, chickpea (garbanzo bean) and quinoa pilaf on page 141.

1 cup fresh coriander (cilantro) leaves

½ cup olive oil

salt and pepper, to taste

1 teaspoon lemon juice

Combine all the ingredients in a blender and blend until smooth and silky.

Refrigerate in an airtight glass container for up to 5 days.

Basil oil

This oil is delicious drizzled over ripe tomatoes as a simple and colourful salad dressing. Slice the tomatoes into rounds, spread on a platter and drizzle this green gold over them. You can spread the tomatoes on a bed of rocket (arugula) or butter lettuce for a simple starter.

1 cup fresh basil leaves

½ cup olive oil

salt and pepper, to taste

1 teaspoon lemon juice

Combine all the ingredients in a blender and blend until smooth and silky.

Refrigerate in an airtight glass container for up to 5 days.

Roasted capsicum (bell pepper) oil

This colourful oil is lovely to look at, and delicious. Use this oil when you need to brighten the vegetables on your plate, or drizzle over a fresh pasta dish just before serving. If you're in a hurry, use a raw capsicum (bell pepper)!

1 roasted red capsicum (bell pepper), skin removed (see page 71)

½ cup olive oil

salt and pepper, to taste

1 teaspoon lemon juice

Combine all the ingredients in a blender and blend until smooth and silky.

Refrigerate in an airtight glass container for up to 5 days.

CURRY BLEND FOR VEGETABLE CURRIES

PREPARATION: 5 MINUTES | MAKES 1 CUP

This is a great basic curry mixture. There is no chilli (chili pepper) in this blend, so feel free to add a little if you enjoy a slight bite to your curries. However, you can always slice up a fresh chilli and allow everyone to choose their own level of heat, after being served.

4 tablespoons
 coriander seeds

1 heaped tablespoon
 sweet paprika

1 heaped tablespoon
 turmeric powder

2 tablespoons cumin seeds

1 heaped tablespoon
 mustard seeds

2 teaspoons fennel seeds

1 teaspoon cinnamon or
 1 cinnamon stick

2 teaspoons ground ginger

½ teaspoon green cardamom
 seeds

In a bowl, combine all the ingredients, stirring well to distribute the seeds evenly.

Store in an airtight container away from light and heat.

When you need a curry powder, simply grind a few tablespoons of this mixture together, being sure to sieve the amount you need through a fine sieve before using, to keep the hard pieces of the spices our of your dish.

Tip
Grinding your own spices allows you to benefit from their fresh flavour, because sitting on grocery-store shelves diminishes the fragrant oils in the seeds over time. Grind the amount you need and then simply add to a hot pan that you've removed from the heat. Stir for 1 minute and then use. The heat allows the oils in the spices to bloom and become more flavourful, but they easily burn, so doing it this way prevents any possible bitter aftertaste.

Turmeric

Turmeric is believed to have originated in India, where it has been used for at least 2500 years. The active component in turmeric is called curcumin (the yellow pigment), which gives it its colour, and it's a very potent antioxidant and anti-inflammatory agent. Due to its unique phytochemical profile, which researchers believe is unique in the world of spices, it has the potential to reverse neuronal damage and may be useful for removing heavy metals from tissues. However, it needs to be consumed with oil in some form, such as coconut oil or cream, because this increases its bioavailability. Adding it to the turmeric macadamia mayonnaise (see recipe on page 72) is a wonderful way to use it regularly and enjoy its brain benefits, as is preparing meals that contain curry powder. Add a sprinkle to smoothies too if you don't find the flavour too overpowering.

FRESH THAI SPICE PASTE

PREPARATION: 15 MINUTES | MAKES 1 CUP

You can use this mixture in stir-fries, green Thai curries with lightly steamed fresh greens, as the basis for a soup, with a few rice or buckwheat noodles and some tofu, or even as a marinade for grilled vegetables; or see page 144 for a recipe that uses this blend. I usually make double or triple of this recipe and store the leftovers in the freezer.

6 fresh kaffir lime leaves (double-leaved), hard spine removed

4 sticks fresh lemongrass, hard outer leaves removed, finely sliced

1 small bunch fresh coriander (cilantro), roughly chopped

2 large garlic cloves

1 tablespoon grated fresh ginger or a 3-centimetre/ 1-inch knob of ginger

1 teaspoon dried ginger

2 teaspoons coconut sugar

1 tablespoon lemon juice

⅓ cup coconut cream

salt, to taste

Combine all the ingredients in a blender, and grind until they form a smooth paste.

Refrigerate in an airtight glass container for up to 5 days.

Variations

Add a can (400 millilitres/13 fluid ounces) of coconut cream to this mixture to make a fragrant sauce to pour over vegetables before oven baking.

Add 1 teaspoon fresh green or red chilli (chili pepper), seeds removed, to add some heat.

Use as a salad dressing by bringing to room temperature and adding a few tablespoons of coconut milk to get it a little runny — especially good on the apple, Chinese cabbage and mint salad (see recipe on page 106).

DUKKAH

PREPARATION 10 MINUTES | MAKES ¾ CUP

This is a nut, seed and spice mixture that has its origins in Egypt, with the word 'dukkah' meaning 'to crush' in the Egyptian Arabic dialect. There are as many different types as the cooks that prepare it, so if you don't have any macadamias use activated almonds or hazelnuts instead, or sunflower seeds instead of sesame seeds. The varieties of spices are also up to you. Serve with gluten-free flat bread (see recipe on page 120) and a small bowl of olive oil.

¼ cup macadamias or almonds

½ cup sesame seeds

2 teaspoon smoked paprika

1 tablespoon lightly roasted coriander (cilantro) seeds

1 tablespoon lightly roasted cumin seeds

1 teaspoon dried thyme leaves

1 teaspoon sea salt

½ teaspoon fresh black pepper

Grind the nuts and seeds together briefly in a food processor, otherwise they will turn into a 'butter'. Transfer to a glass bowl.

Grind the spices and thyme together in the same food processor bowl, then stir into the nut mixture. Add the salt and pepper and stir the mixture.

Refrigerate the mixture in an airtight glass container for up to 2 weeks.

Tip
Sprinkle over salads (see recipes on pages 89–117) for extra flavour and nutrients.

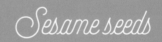
Sesame seeds

Sesame seeds are one of the oldest cultivated crops in the world, having been around for some 4000 years.

Cleopatra is believed to have used sesame oil for her skin. Each seed pod contains 50-100 red, brown, yellow or black seeds. The magical phrase 'Open sesame!' has its origins in the fact that the seed pods shatter at the slightest touch when ripe, sending the seed to the wind, so most of the sesame grown is harvested by hand. Sesamin found in these seeds is a powerful antioxidant and inhibits the production of cholesterol. Whole seeds contain 18 per cent protein and 10 times the amount of calcium as milk, including magnesium, manganese, selenium, iron and zinc, as well as the antioxidant vitamin E. Tahini, made from crushed sesame seeds, is 45 per cent protein and 55 per cent oil. Use unhulled tahini, which contains lignins that are helpful hormone balancers. They do not contain any omega-3 but do contain 45 per cent omega-6, the rest being omega-9. Tahini is a nutrient-dense brain food.

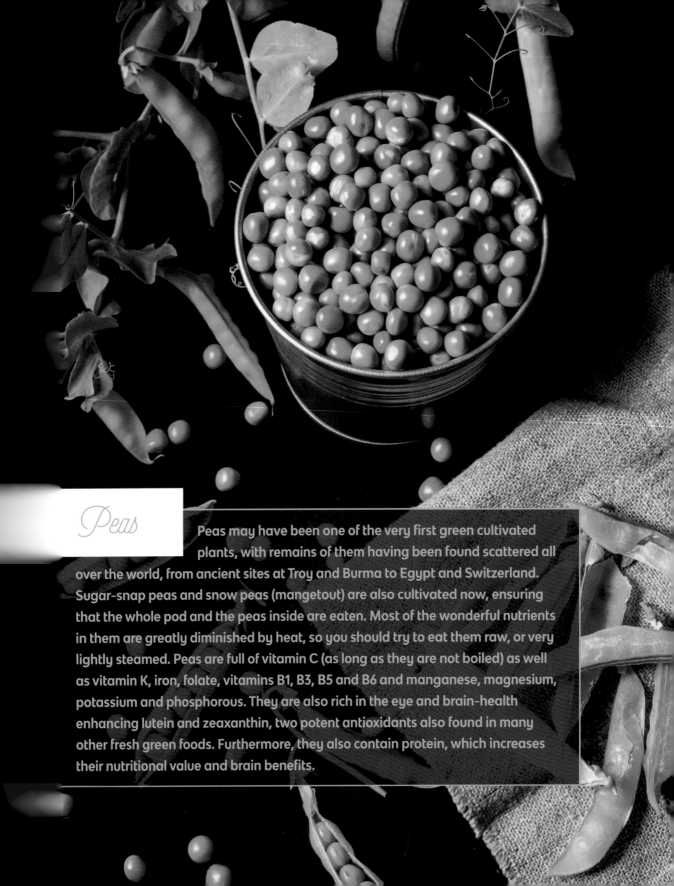

Peas

Peas may have been one of the very first green cultivated plants, with remains of them having been found scattered all over the world, from ancient sites at Troy and Burma to Egypt and Switzerland. Sugar-snap peas and snow peas (mangetout) are also cultivated now, ensuring that the whole pod and the peas inside are eaten. Most of the wonderful nutrients in them are greatly diminished by heat, so you should try to eat them raw, or very lightly steamed. Peas are full of vitamin C (as long as they are not boiled) as well as vitamin K, iron, folate, vitamins B1, B3, B5 and B6 and manganese, magnesium, potassium and phosphorous. They are also rich in the eye and brain-health enhancing lutein and zeaxanthin, two potent antioxidants also found in many other fresh green foods. Furthermore, they also contain protein, which increases their nutritional value and brain benefits.

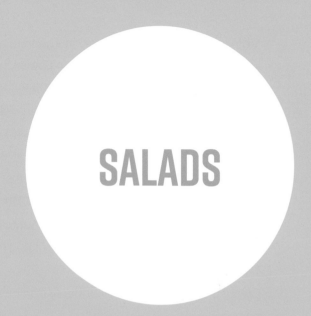

SALADS

It is entirely possible to prepare and eat such a wide variety of different salads that eating them every day never bores you. By simply adding a different vegetable, and dressing, you create a different flavour. Salads can also be either side dishes or transformed into main meals by the simple addition of some legumes or quinoa. Washing and preparing your salad ingredients is made simple today by the 'washed and ready to eat' packs of lettuce, herbs and sprouts available for purchase, although none of them can compare with fresh greens from your local organic market (or your own garden!). There are also so many different vegetables available today that one is spoilt for choice when preparing great-tasting salads. Remember to always make extra salad in the evening because it's the best leftover lunch ever.

Remember the following when preparing salads.

- Dress salads just before serving — doing so long before serving means that everything goes limp. Alternatively, simply pour the dressing into the bottom of the salad bowl, add the lettuce and then just toss before serving. I like to keep my dressing separate because then it's much easier to use the leftovers for lunch the next day because the salad stays crisp and fresh.

- The best salads are often the simplest — with just three or four ingredients and a stunning dressing.

- Main-course salads are bulkier and generally contain some legumes, such as kidney beans, chickpeas (garbanzo beans), nuts or seeds, or can be a salad based on a grain of choice, my favourite being quinoa.

- Side salads should complement the main dish — don't add tomatoes to the salad if the main course is tomato-based. And serve crunchy, herb-filled salads with creamy dishes.

- A salad dressing should enhance the taste of a salad, not disguise it. Choose heavy, creamy dressings for sturdy salad leaves, and light dressings for delicate leaves.

- Think about the texture of a salad — too much crunch and everyone's jaws will ache; too little crunch and it seems as if you're eating air. Balance the crunch, especially for children.

- Colour is very important in salads, so don't over-use it. We eat with our eyes too.

- Tearing large leaves to the same size as smaller leaves will ensure that salad leaves do not have to be cut on your plate and the dressing is evenly distributed on all leaves when it is added.

Remember to ...

- Sprinkle lemon rind over salads to get a 'hit' of sunshine and sparkle (see page 15).

- Sprinkle 'marinated' red onion over salads (see page 16) for a glorious colour and nutrients.

- Toss a few tablespoons of the sun-dried tomatoes you prepared in advance into salads (see page 15).

- Sprinkle the beetroot (beet) prepared in advance (see page 15) into salads just before serving.

- Sprinkle a few tablespoons of quinoa (see page 29) over any leafy salads to increase nutrient density.

- Use nuts and seeds sprinkled over any salad to add both crunch and nutrients.

- Use sprouts on any salads — they enhance the nutritional value and add great crunch appeal. Making your own means that you have an endless supply of these great nutrient-dense salad toppings.

- You can easily transform pesto into a salad dressing if you don't have time to whip up a new one. Simply combine some pesto with some lemon juice, olive oil and a dash of herb salt and you can drizzle this over your salad.

Experimenting with different varieties of lettuce and other green leaves provides you with a huge range of flavours and textures — and nutrients.

- Choose cos (romaine) or iceberg leaves when you want a crunchy salad with texture and bulk. Serve these lettuce types alone, because they will overpower more delicate leaves.
- Choose frisée (curly endive), chicory (endive) or radicchio for a salad that needs some bitter leaves. These lettuce leaves provide an interesting contrast of flavours when they are mixed with the peppery lettuce or leaf greens, such as rocket (arugula).
- Choose rocket (arugula), watercress, mustard and cress for peppery flavours in salads. They are feisty and flavoursome — eat them on their own or mix them with soft and bitter leaves.
- Choose baby spinach, lamb's lettuce or lollo rosso (red leaf lettuce) when you need a bulky salad, which can be perked up with some peppery or herb leaves.

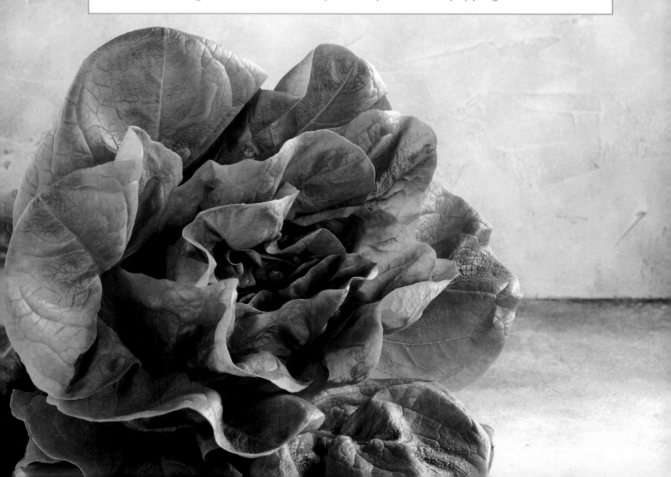

SUPER-FAST GOLDEN COLESLAW

PREPARATION TIME: 20 MINUTES | SERVES 6–8

Coleslaw is one of my favourite salads, and I think it's because I love creamy, lemony, salad dressings. But store-bought mayonnaise is not filled with brain-friendly ingredients, and it is really simple to make your own, if you know the basics. Use the turmeric macadamia mayonnaise recipe from page 72. Adding fresh coriander (cilantro) helps the salad become even more brain friendly, because coriander may be a very effective mercury detoxifier, a heavy metal that is particularly damaging to brain tissue. I use a mandolin to slice my cabbage and the leek into fine strips but prefer to slice the carrots into thin julienne strips. The various textures add interest and crunch to the salad, while the creamy mayonnaise adds great mouthfeel.

4 cups finely sliced cabbage

1 small leek, finely sliced — and rinsed well to ensure there is no sand present

2 medium carrots, grated (a combination of orange and yellow carrots works well)

1 yellow/orange beetroot (golden beet), grated (optional)

1 bunch fresh coriander (cilantro), washed well and chopped finely, leaving a few leaves for serving

In a large bowl, combine all the ingredients. Toss with the turmeric macadamia mayonnaise (see recipe on page 72) and serve immediately with a few sprigs of coriander (cilantro) to garnish.

Variations

Toss with 1 cup activated pecans, roughly chopped, for extra nutrients.

Add 1 tablespoon curry powder (see recipe on page 85) to the mayonnaise before tossing through the salad for a 'curry' coleslaw.

Beetroot

Beetroot (beet) has been cultivated since prehistoric times and was originally grown for its leaves. It is the descendant of the wild sea beet, which is native to the coasts of southern Asia, northern Africa and Europe. The Romans and Greeks, who reserved the roots for medicinal purposes, mainly for blood and digestion-related ailments, ate the green leaves. They are an excellent provider of potassium, iron, magnesium and manganese, with the leaves being high in vitamins A and C, as well as calcium, folic acid and iron, all good brain nutrients. Use the leaves in salads — the smaller leaves are tastier (and less fibrous) than the large ones.

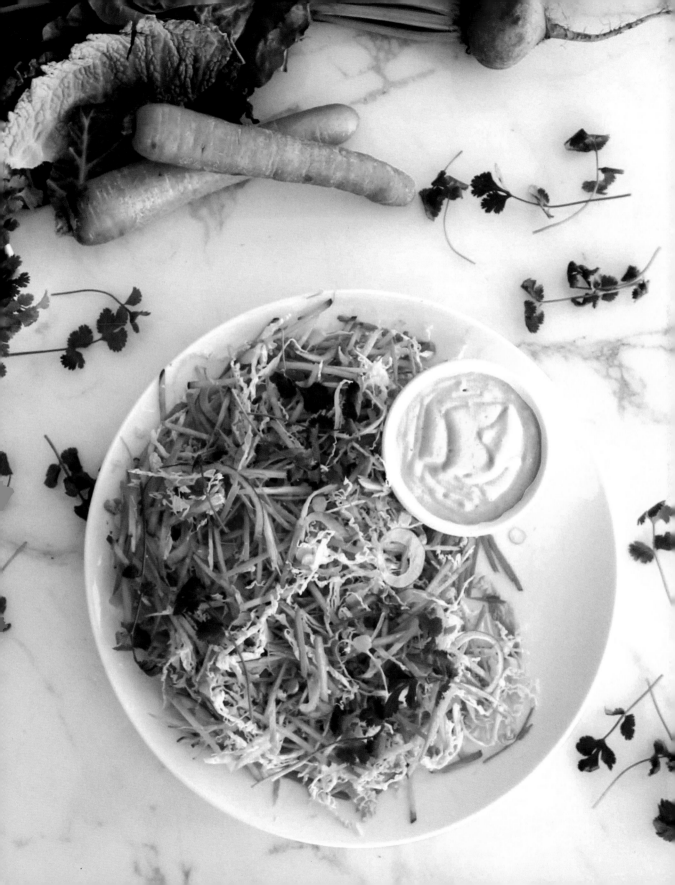

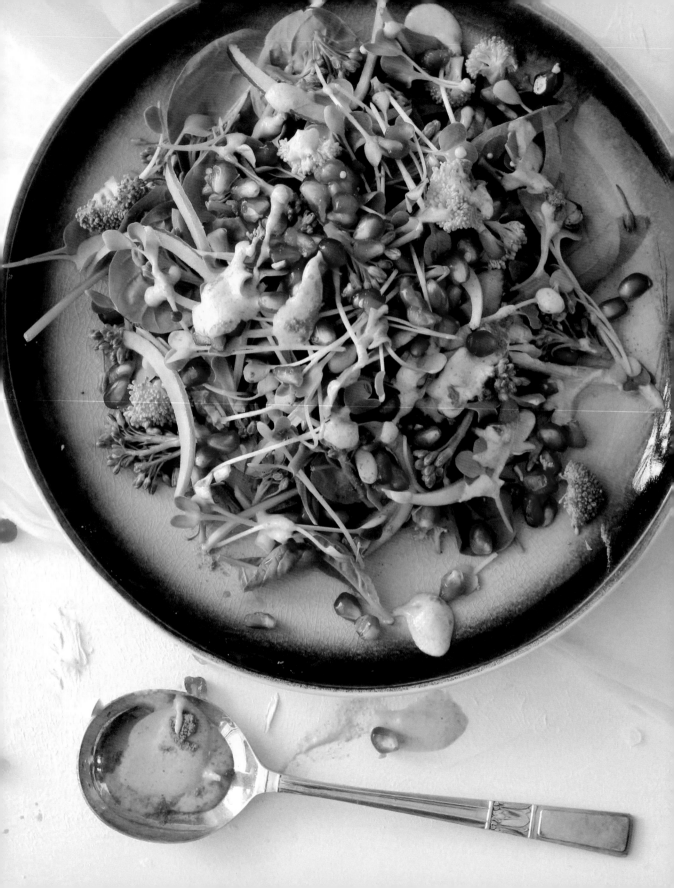

BROCCOLI AND POMEGRANATE SALAD

PREPARATION: 15 MINUTES | SERVES 6–8

This is a beautiful-looking salad, and one that will become nutrient dense if you accompany it with one of the salad dressings from pages 66–72, especially the turmeric macadamia mayonnaise.

1 head broccoli, broken into small florets and sliced in half

3–4 cups baby spinach or small lettuce leaves, broken into bite-sized pieces

½ red onion, peeled and finely sliced

2 cups fresh sprouts — sunflower or radish if you want a slight 'warm bite'

1 large pomegranate, peeled, seeded (retain half the seeds to sprinkle over the salad just before serving)

2–3 small spring onions (shallots, scallions), finely sliced

Lightly steam the broccoli over boiling water for a few minutes until the florets turn bright green. Remove from the heat and spread on a plate to cool.

In a bowl, combine the spinach leaves, onion, sprouts and pomegranate flesh, and toss well. Add the cooled broccoli and toss through the other ingredients. Sprinkle the pomegranate seeds and spring onions over the top of the salad, and serve with any of the salad dressings from pages 66–72, although I love it with the turmeric macadamia mayonnaise (see recipe on page 72) — the colours and flavour are gorgeous!

Variation

Replace the spinach or lettuce with watercress.

Pomegranate

Pomegranates are one of the oldest fruits known to man. They are native to southeastern Europe and Asia and moved with Spanish missionaries into Mexico and California in the 16th century. The name is derived from the French 'pomme garnet,' and means 'many seeded apple'. It's been a symbol of fertility since ancient times and the Egyptians revered them as symbols of prosperity. Early Christians used this fruit in art to symbolize Christ's resurrection and rebirth. The beautiful reddish/pink colour in the abundant fruit-filled sacs is home to powerful phytonutrients and antioxidants along with possible anti-inflammatory compounds. They also contain brain-friendly potassium, magnesium, phosphorous, iron and zinc. Choose fresh fruit instead of juices that contain lots of sugar.

GORGEOUS GREEN GARDEN SALAD

PREPARATION: 15 MINUTES | SERVES 4–6

The combination of these greens results in a luscious, vibrant salad that shouts, 'Eat me!' When making this for a special meal, ensure you have a roasted garlic head (see page 70) to squeeze over the steamed greens before tossing them with the other greens. Use any salad dressing of your choice, although the tomato salad cream (see recipe on page 67) works very well. Mustard sprouts, with their slight peppery bite, are great and tossing in a chopped avocado just before serving works beautifully too.

2 cups green beans

2 cups broccoli florets

1 head garlic, roasted
 (see page 70)

1 bunch coriander (cilantro),
 finely chopped

1 cup sprouts

1 cup snow pea (mangetout)
 sprouts

1 large cucumber, thinly sliced

1⅓ cups or 1 can
 (425 grams/15 ounces)
 chickpeas (garbanzo beans),
 drained

½ cup pine nuts

Steam the beans and broccoli over boiling water for a few minutes, so as to retain their bright green colour, nutrients and crunch. Set the greens aside, squeeze the garlic over them and allow them to cool slightly while you prepare the rest of the salad.

Meanwhile, in a large bowl, combine the coriander, sprouts, cucumber and chickpeas, and toss well.

Toss the garlicky greens through the rest of the salad, then top with the pine nuts and serve with your dressing of choice on the side.

Variation
Sprinkle ½ teaspoon of turmeric on the dressing before serving to add a hit of antioxidant power.

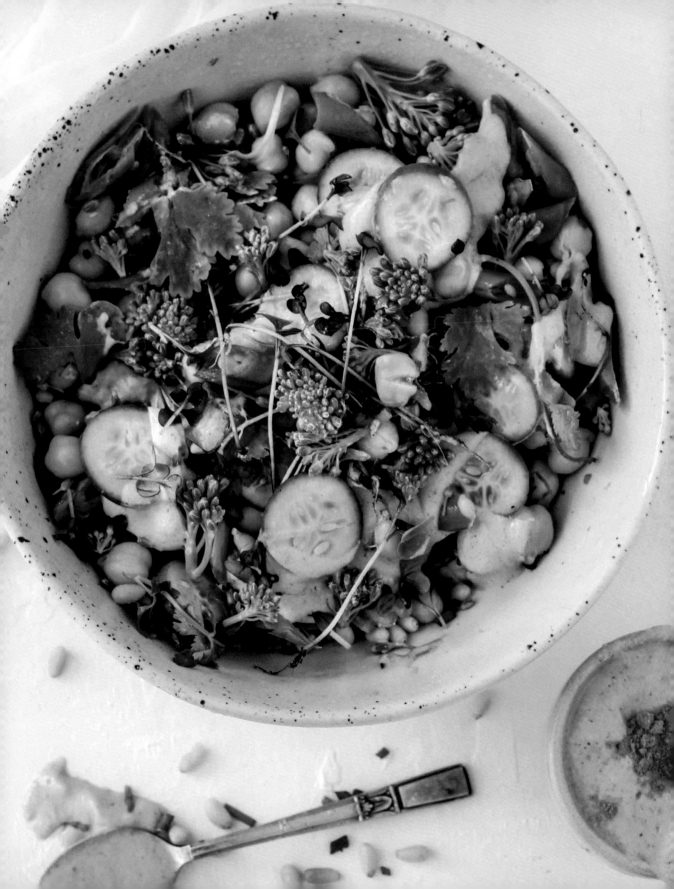

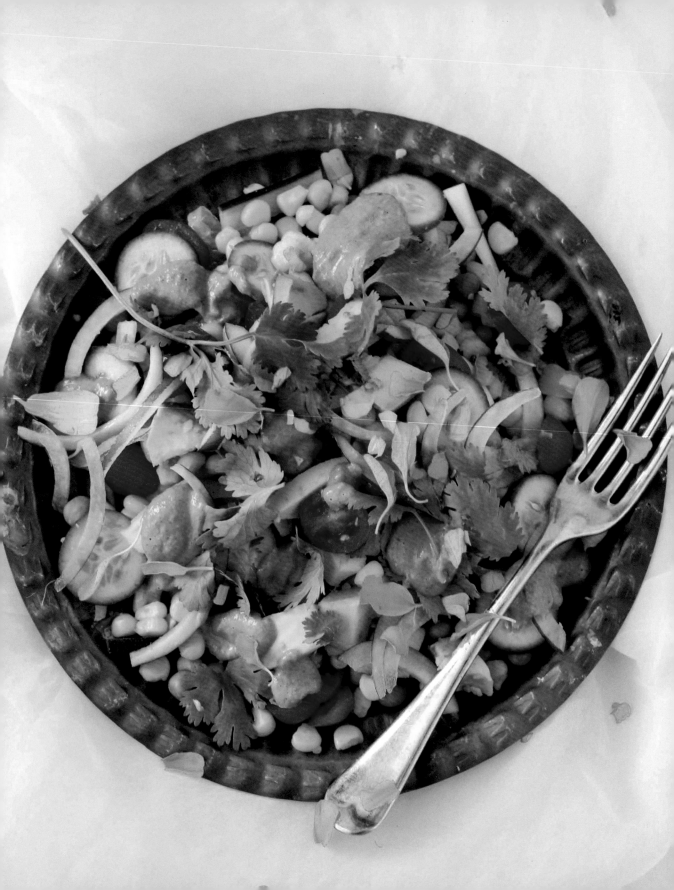

SWEET CORN, PEA AND CORIANDER (CILANTRO) SALAD

PREPARATION: 15 MINUTES | SERVES 4-6

We had some fresh sweet corn, lovely ripe avocados, fresh peas and fresh coriander (cilantro), so we decided to toss it all together for this simple salad — the result was quite delicious. The bright yellow and green result also looks amazing. You could easily use fresh basil — it would work just as well — although in that case I would add small, ripe cherry tomatoes. The roasted red capsicum (bell pepper) salad dressing (see recipe on page 71) or the tomato salad cream dressing (see recipe on page 67) both work well here, enhancing the colour and flavour.

1 cup sweet corn (frozen or fresh and chopped off the cob)

1 cup peas (frozen or fresh)

1 cucumber, sliced into matchsticks

1 medium red onion, peeled and finely sliced

1 avocado, diced

handful of cherry tomatoes, halved

1 small bunch fresh coriander (cilantro), finely sliced

Lightly steam the corn and peas over boiling water for 5 minutes and then remove from the heat and cool on a large plate.

Over a sieve, drain the liquid off the cucumber sticks.

In a large bowl, combine the remaining salad ingredients. Add the corn and peas and toss together, then toss in the drained cucumber sticks. Serve immediately with the salad dressing on the side.

Variation
Replace the coriander with finely sliced fresh basil leaves.

Tip
Flower petals can add colour and interest to salads — just make completely sure they are pesticide free and edible, and don't add too many, because some petals can be quite spicy. Use the flowers of chives, garlic and leeks, as well as borage, calendula/marigold, carnation and jasmine petals. Chamomile flowers, along with coriander (cilantro) and dill flowers, are pretty and tasty, while citrus blossoms are highly scented and can be overpowering.

GREEN AND WHITE SALAD

PREPARATION: 15 MINUTES | SERVES 4–6

This is a really simple salad — just choose whichever of the following vegetables you have on hand — five or six — in the quantity you need. Serve with either the raspberry salad dressing (see recipe on page 67), the tomato salad cream (see recipe on page 67), the tahini herb dressing (see recipe on page 66) or the mango mustard salad dressing (see recipe on page 66). They are all very tasty!

½ head broccoli, finely sliced

20 spears fresh asparagus, finely sliced horizontally

1 large handful sugar-snap peas, cut into horizontal matchsticks

½ butter lettuce, roughly broken into pieces

10–15 button mushrooms, wiped and finely sliced

1 small bunch rocket (arugula), roughly broken into strips

1 small bunch spring onions (shallots, scallions), finely chopped

1 cup sprouts

1 zucchini (courgette), finely sliced

1 small bunch watercress, broken into bite-sized pieces

Steam the broccoli, asparagus and sugar-snap peas over boiling water for a few minutes, so as to retain their bright green colour, nutrients and crunch. Set the greens aside to cool.

Meanwhile, in a large bowl, combine the remaining ingredients, then toss the greens through the salad.

Variations

Sprinkle pumpkin seeds (pepitas) or sunflower seeds over the salad before serving.

If using the tahini dressing or turmeric macadamia mayonnaise, sprinkle pomegranate seeds over the salad before serving.

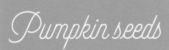

Pumpkin seeds

The oldest evidence of pumpkin seeds (pepitas) dates back to between 7000 and 5500 BC in Mexico. They are high in magnesium and zinc, as well as iron, manganese and potassium. They are also a good source of protein, and contain a wide array of the various forms of vitamin E, which are potent antioxidants, very helpful for our busy, energy-producing brains.

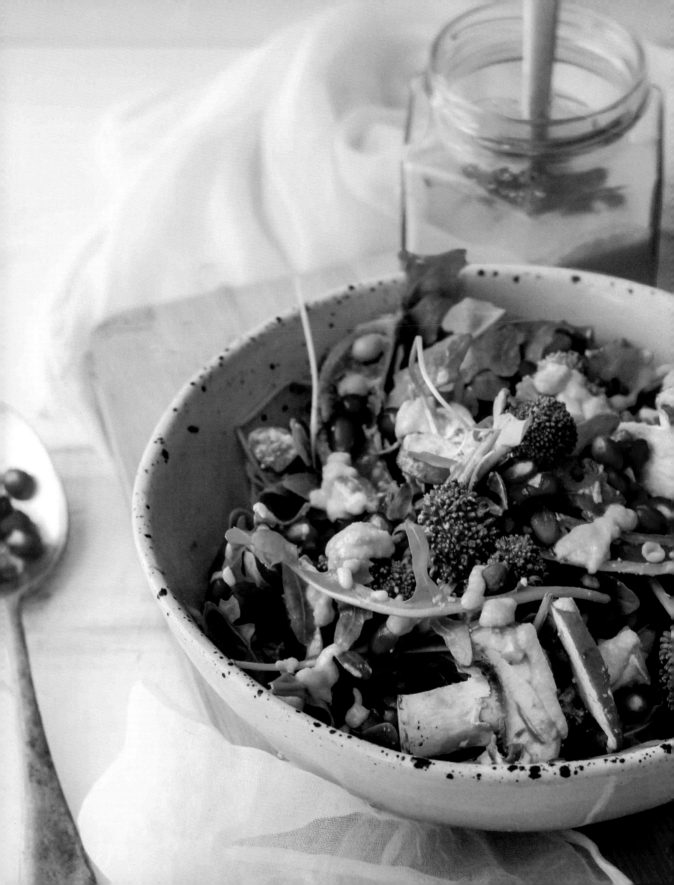

SUPERFOOD SALAD

PREPARATION: 45 MINUTES | SERVES 4–6

The superfoods in this recipe are: quinoa, baby kale, avocado and pomegranate seeds. Quinoa makes a great base for a salad because it's chewy, nutty and full of protein and fibre. Serve with any of the salad dressings from page 66–72, although the tahini herb and the tomato salad cream dressings are especially lovely with this salad.

1 cup cooked quinoa
(see page 29)

2 cups baby kale, chopped
into bite-sized pieces

1 large garlic clove, peeled
and crushed

juice of 1 lemon (and rind, as
per variation below)

¼ cup olive oil

½ teaspoon herb salt

1 cup pomegranate seeds
(retain a few to sprinkle over
the salad to serve)

1 avocado, chopped

5 spring onions (shallots,
scallions), including green
stems, finely sliced

Place the cooked quinoa in a large bowl to cool.

In a separate bowl, combine the kale, garlic, lemon juice, olive oil and herb salt. Massage the kale well with your hands to disperse the seasonings and soften the leaves.

Add the kale mixture to the quinoa and then the pomegranate seeds, avocado and spring onion and toss well.

You can serve immediately with a dressing of your choice or make this salad a day ahead and refrigerate overnight in an airtight glass container.

Variations

Toss in a handful of finely chopped coriander (cilantro) and the rind of a lemon.

Toss in 1–2 cups cooked spicy sweet potato cubes (page 16) to turn this salad into a main meal.

Sprinkle with a handful of hemp seeds to add extra nutrients and essential fatty acids.

Hemp seeds

Misleading information has surrounded hemp with mystery, due to the mistaken belief that eating hemp seeds will have the same effect as smoking the leaves of their distant cousin, the marijuana plant. There are about 2000 different varieties of cannabis plants, with 90 per cent of them being harmless and the remaining 10 per cent having high levels of tetrahydrocannabinol (THC). They are very nutrient dense seeds, containing 20 per cent omega-3, 60 per cent omega-6 and 12 per cent omega-9. They also contain protein and a number of B vitamins, vitamins E and D, magnesium, iron and zinc, making them a great brain food.

RAINBOW NOODLE SALAD WITH MAYONNAISE (RECIPE CONTINUES OVERLEAF)

PREPARATION: 30 MINUTES | SERVES 6–8

The lovely thing about this salad is that it is very easy to make, and can easily be transformed into rice paper rolls. Then all you have to do is serve them with a few bowls of mayonnaise, sweet chilli sauce and plain tamari soya (soy) sauce.

Salad

1 small bunch coriander (cilantro)

1 small bunch mint

1 cup frozen peas

1 cup frozen sweet corn

1 packet (approximately 200–250 grams/7–9 ounces) rice vermicelli or 1 packet buckwheat noodles

2 large carrots, peeled and grated

½ Chinese cabbage, finely sliced

1 small red onion, peeled and finely sliced

2 sticks celery, finely sliced

1 small red capsicum (bell pepper), finely sliced

½ cup unsalted peanuts or ½ cup whole cashew nuts

Dressing

½ cup cashew nuts or macadamia nuts

1 large garlic clove

¼ teaspoon ground ginger or 1 small knob fresh ginger

¼ teaspoon cumin seeds

¼ teaspoon coriander (cilantro) seeds

⅛ cup tamari soya (soy) sauce

juice of 1 medium lemon

½ cup olive oil

3 ice cubes

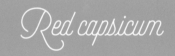

Red capsicums (bell peppers) are native to Mexico, Central and Northern South America, where 2000-year-old remains have been found. They contain significant amounts of vitamin C (actually three times the amount contained in oranges), B5 and B6, vitamins E and K and beta-carotene, being converted into vitamin A. They also contain calcium, phosphorus and iron, as well as magnesium and manganese, and lutein, the 'brain and eye' antioxidant, along with a less-known phytonutrient called beta-cryptoxanthin.

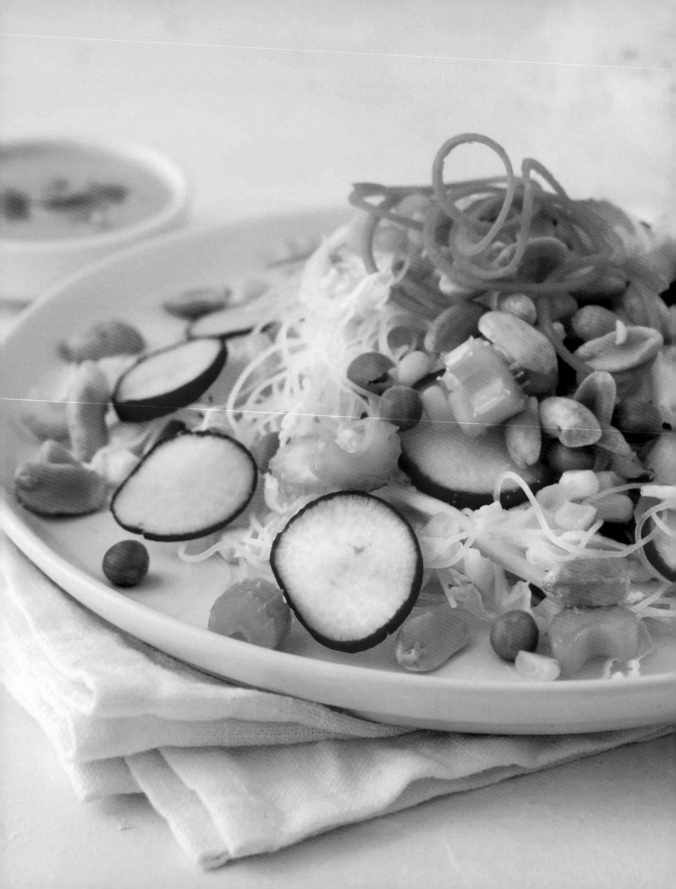

RAINBOW NOODLE SALAD WITH MAYONNAISE (CONTINUED)

To make the salad, thoroughly wash the fresh coriander leaves and mint, then finely slice both. Set aside most of the herbs to use in the salad, and a small amount of each to use as a garnish.

Lightly steam the peas and sweet corn over boiling water for 5 minutes, then set aside.

Meanwhile, prepare the noodles according to the packet instructions. Drain the noodles well, otherwise the salad will be soggy, and use kitchen scissors to chop them into pieces. Transfer them to a large bowl and add the carrot, cabbage, onion, celery and capsicum. Add the fresh coriander, mint, peas and sweet corn, and set aside while you prepare the dressing.

To make the dressing, combine all the dressing ingredients in a blender and blend until they form a smooth, creamy mayonnaise. This will take about 60 seconds. Transfer to a jug.

Sprinkle the nuts over the salad and serve with the dressing on the side.

Variations

Instead of the salad dressing above, use the peanut satay sauce on page 78.

If you would like to turn this into a simple stir-fry, toss all the salad ingredients into a hot wok for a few minutes until heated through, which will leave the vegetables crunchy and lightly cooked, and serve with the peanut satay sauce on page 78.

Toss in the baked tofu from page 116 to increase the nutrient density and the size of this dish.

Tip

Sweet chilli sauce is very simple to make. Simply finely chop a small chilli (chili pepper), taking care not to touch your eyes until you have finished chopping and washed your hands thoroughly. Remove the seeds if you want the mixture to be mild, and add 2 tablespoons of real maple or rice syrup, the juice of ¼ lemon, a pinch of salt and a tablespoon of olive oil to the chilli slices. Stir well to combine and serve as a dipping sauce to rice paper rolls.

APPLE, CHINESE CABBAGE AND MINT SALAD

PREPARATION: 20 MINUTES | SERVES 6

This is a wonderfully fresh, crunchy salad. The apples and mint combine beautifully to produce an attractive start to a meal, as well as providing loads of enzymes and antioxidants. Serve with any of the dressings from pages 66–72, although the coriander (cilantro) and pine nut mayonnaise (see recipe on page 69) is especially lovely with this salad, as is a dollop of the Thai paste diluted slightly with coconut milk (see recipe on page 86)

4 green apples, sliced into julienne sticks

2 large avocados, peeled and sliced into slivers

1 small lemon

½ Chinese cabbage, thinly sliced

1 leek, thinly sliced, or 5–6 spring onions (shallots, scallions), thinly sliced

1 bunch mint, washed carefully and leaves separated and put aside

1 bunch coriander (cilantro), washed carefully and set aside

1 cup pistachio nuts, shelled

In a large bowl, combine the apple and avocado, and squeeze the lemon juice over to stop them discolouring while you prepare the rest of the salad.

Add the cabbage and leek or spring onion. Top with the mint, coriander and pistachios just before serving.

Variation
Add 1 cup grated carrot and 1 cup grated beetroot (beet), and replace the pistachios with walnuts.

Apple remains have been found dating as far back as 6500 BC in the Jordan Valley and are believed to have originated in the mountainside border between Kazakhstan and northwest China but are now grown globally. The custom of giving a teacher an apple originated when a community paid whatever they could afford. Apples contain the antioxidants quercetin and epicatechin (also found in green tea.) They also contain chromium, which helps keep blood sugar levels stable, which brain cells appreciate. They contain fibre in the form of pectin and vitamin C. The average conventionally grown apple has between 20 and 30 artificial poisons on its skin, so choosing organic apples is the healthiest way to enjoy these fruits.

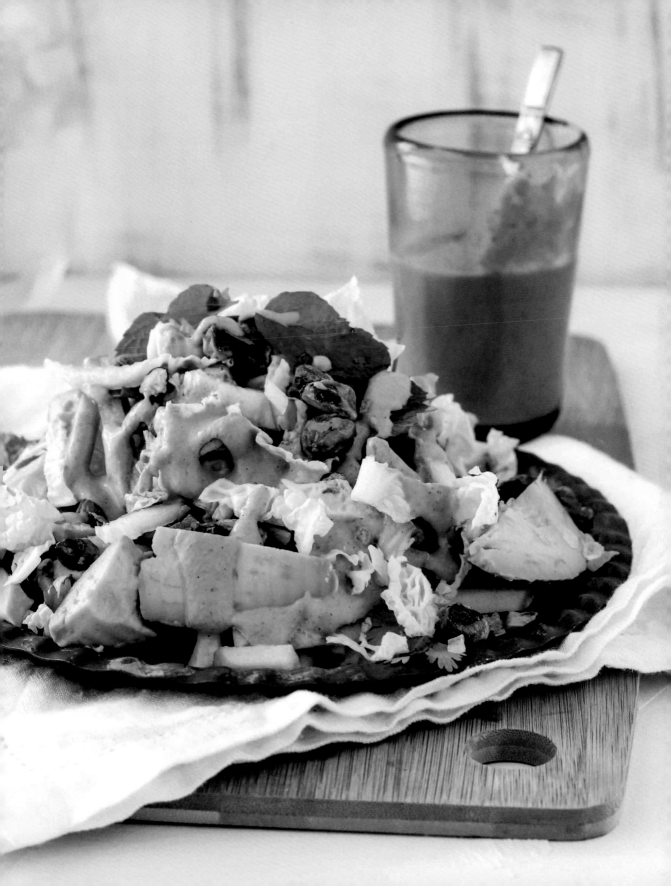

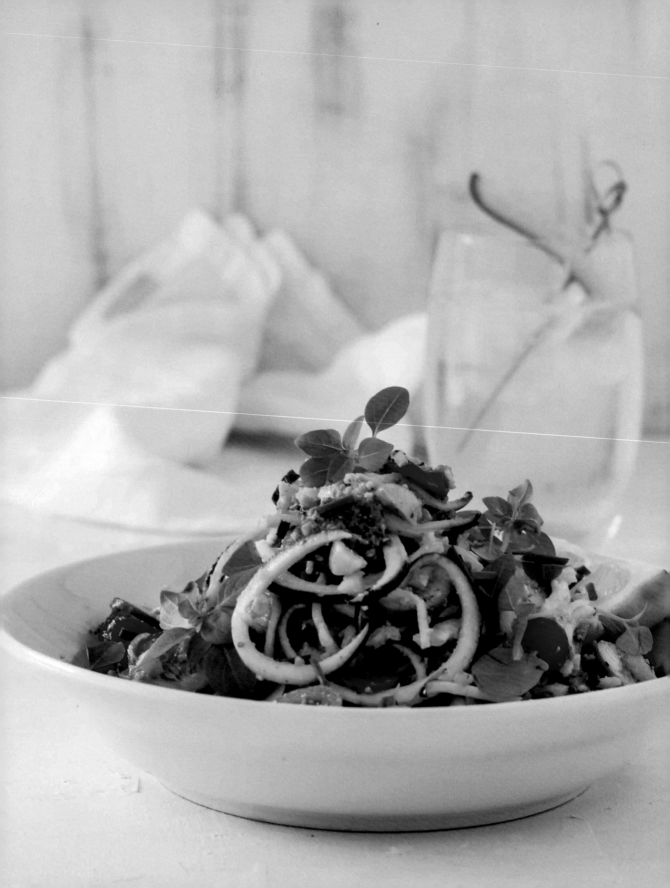

ZUCCHINI (COURGETTE), CUCUMBER AND TOMATO SALAD

PREPARATION: 20 MINUTES | SERVES 4–6

Spiralized zucchini 'pasta' has been very popular for a number of years, but if you don't own a spiralizer you don't have to miss out on this tasty way to eat zucchini. I use my mandolin to grate the zucchini, but you can use an ordinary grater too. The only challenge with this salad is that it tends to get soggy if you make it too far in advance of eating it, and it is therefore also not a good leftover salad the next day. However, it's a really fresh and vibrant salad and you can make extra to serve as a main-course 'pasta' dish too. With both pesto and macadamia nuts, it is also very satisfying.

3 zucchini (courgette), washed, top and bottom cut off and spiralized, julienned or grated

3 spring onions (shallots, scallions), finely sliced

half a head of small lettuce, finely sliced

1 Lebanese or short cucumber, finely sliced

squeeze of lemon

1 cup baby tomatoes, quartered

¼ cup green pesto (see recipe on page 73)

¼ cup of coriander (cilantro) or basil, finely sliced

½ cup macadamia nuts, roughly chopped

salt, to taste

Prepare the zucchini according to your choice, and transfer to a colander, pressing down lightly to remove excess moisture.

In a large bowl, combine the remaining ingredients and then add the zucchini, tossing carefully to coat with the pesto.

Variations

Replace the zucchini with 2 carrots and toss in a handful of finely chopped mint leaves.

Replace the fresh tomatoes with ½ cup prepared sun-dried tomatoes (see page 16).

Sprinkle a few tablespoons of hemp seeds over the salad just before serving.

ROASTED CAULIFLOWER AND DILL SALAD

PREPARATION: 20 MINUTES | SERVES 6

This is a very simple salad to make when you have taken care of baking the cauliflower and if you have a salad dressing ready. Feel free to use any of the salad dressings in this book, although the instant mayonnaise (see recipe on page 68) is especially good.

1 cauliflower, washed and broken into florets

5–6 spring onions (shallots, scallions), finely sliced

3–4 cups baby kale leaves, washed and drained

1 cup celery, finely sliced

¼ cup fresh dill, finely chopped

olive oil

Preheat the oven to 160°C/320°F. Line a baking tray with baking paper.

Spread the cauliflower florets evenly over the baking sheet. Bake for 8–10 minutes, until they are tender when you insert a sharp knife into a stalk, then remove from the oven and spread on a platter to cool slightly, sprinkling with the olive oil.

In a large bowl, combine the remaining ingredients and toss well.

Toss the cauliflower into the salad and serve immediately with any of the dressings from pages 66–72.

Variation
To transform this salad into a light meal, add a drained can (425 grams/15 ounces) of lentils or 1⅓ cups cooked lentils to the salad ingredients before adding the cauliflower.

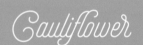

Cauliflower

Cauliflower originated in China and then moved to the Middle East. The Moors introduced it to Spain in the 12th century and it found its way to England via the established trade routes of the time. It is a member of the cabbage family. The word cauliflower comes from two Latin terms and literally means 'cabbage flower'. The earliest cauliflowers were the size of tennis balls, but they have been cultivated to the enormous sizes we see today. The phyto-chemicals found in these cruciferous vegetables (namely cabbages, broccoli, cauliflower, Brussels sprouts, watercress, turnips, kale, pak choi (bok choy), mustard greens, chard, swede (rutabaga) and spring greens) are invaluable in stimulating the body's enzyme defences against carcinogens. They also contain potassium, iron and zinc, all important brain nutrients. They also contain the antioxidants vitamins A and C, although cooking does reduce their presence.

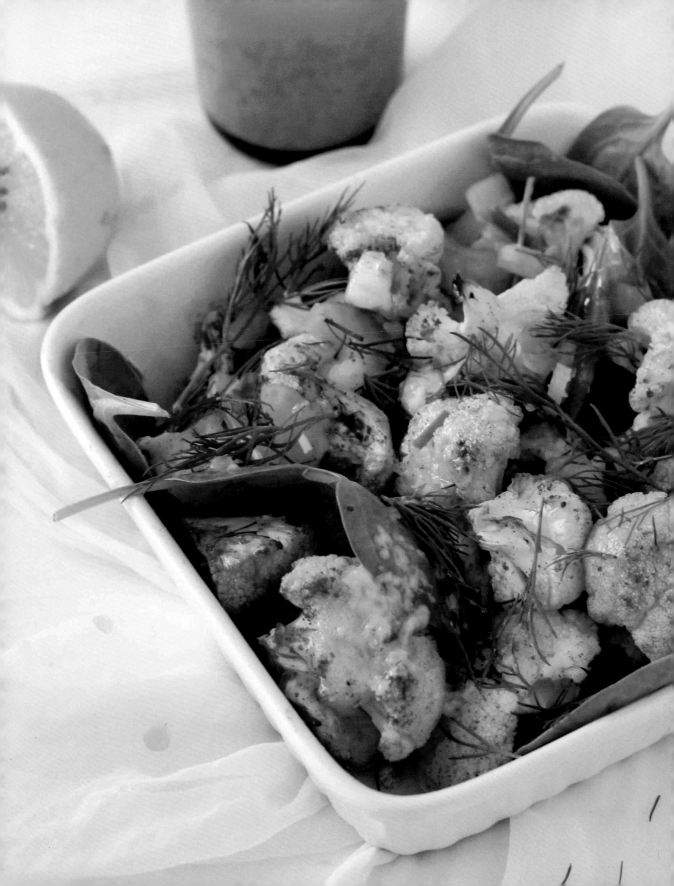

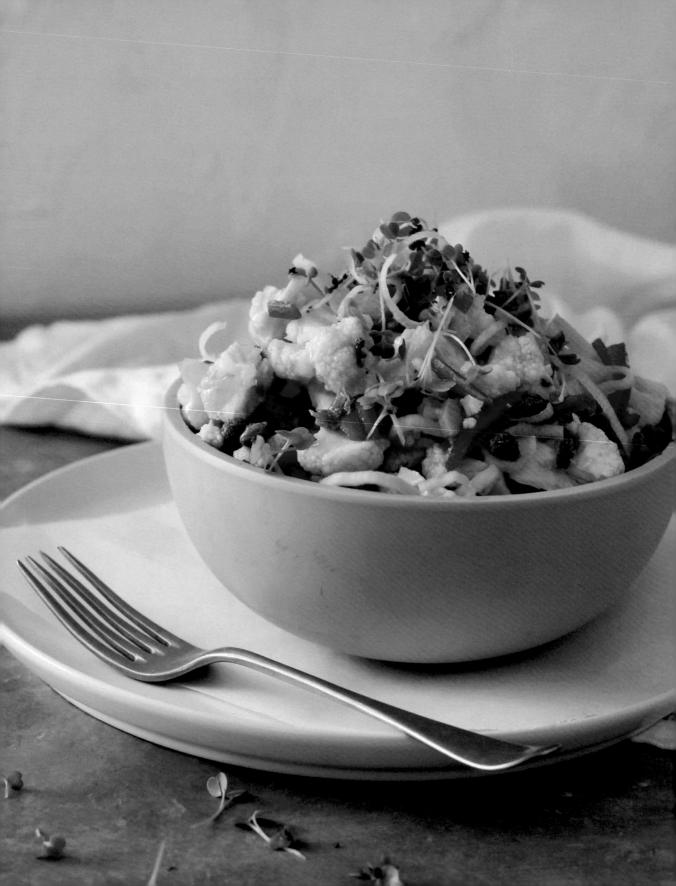

MARINATED CAULIFLOWER AND RED CAPSICUM (BELL PEPPER) SALAD

PREPARATION: 20 MINUTES | SERVES 6

This is a very simple but satisfying salad, and serving it with the gluten-free flat bread (see recipe on page 120) and red capsicum (bell pepper) hummus (see recipe on page 75) makes for an ideal light meal. It's also a really pretty salad and looks lovely spread out on a bed of baby spinach or rocket (arugula) leaves topped with either of the roasted garlic dressings on pages 70 and 71.

Salad

1 medium cauliflower, stem removed and florets thinly sliced

1 small leek, finely sliced

1 red capsicum (bell pepper), seeded and finely sliced

Dressing

juice and rind of 1 medium lemon

1 tablespoon mustard powder

½ cup olive oil

3 tablespoons maple syrup

4 tablespoons capers, rinsed and drained

½ cup parsley or coriander (cilantro), finely sliced

2 spring onions (shallots, scallions), finely chopped (including green tops)

rind of 1 medium lemon

Steam the cauliflower lightly, maintaining a slight crunch, and set aside to cool.

Meanwhile, combine the lemon juice, mustard powder, olive oil and maple syrup in a blender or food processor and blend on high until smooth and creamy. Add the capers and pulse briefly to chop them roughly.

Transfer the mixture to a large bowl, then add the lemon rind, steamed cauliflower, parsley or coriander and spring onion. Toss evenly, then pour the dressing over the salad to serve.

If you don't plan to serve the salad immediately, set aside the parsley or coriander and spring onion. You can refrigerate the salad in an airtight glass container for a few hours or overnight, then return to room temperature and toss the parsley or coriander and spring onions into the salad just before serving so that they retain their colour and crunch.

Variation

Add a drained can (425 grams/15 ounces) or 1⅓ cups cooked chickpeas (garbanzo beans) to transform this salad into a light meal.

SPICY WARM LENTIL, APRICOT AND PINE NUT SALAD

PREPARATION: 40 MINUTES | SERVES 4–6

This spicy lentil salad can make a filling main meal if coupled with some crusty bread (see flat bread recipe on page 120). It is filling and tasty — the cumin lends an exotic touch, while the apricot slivers and pine nuts add richness. If you can't find any pine nuts, use the variations below. If you make this salad a few hours ahead of time the flavours intensify. I serve this salad on a bed of fresh baby spinach leaves, watercress, rocket (arugula) or a variety of lettuce leaves.

1 large onion, peeled and quartered

½ cup dried apricots, finely sliced

2–3 spring onions (shallots, scallions), finely chopped

juice and rind of 1 large lemon

3 tablespoons olive oil

salt and pepper, to taste

2 teaspoons ground cumin

2 teaspoons ground coriander

1 large punnet (or 2 cups) mushrooms, rinsed well and sliced

2⅔ cups cooked lentils, or 2 cans (425 grams/15 ounces each) lentils, drained

⅔ cup fresh pine nuts

½ cup fresh coriander (cilantro) or Italian flat-leaf parsley, finely chopped

2 cups green leaves, to serve

1 avocado, peeled and sliced, to serve

Preheat the oven to 180°C/355°F. Line a baking tray with baking paper.

Place the onion quarters on the tray and bake for about 45 minutes. (You can leave the onions out and move onto step three below.) Remove from the oven and set aside.

Meanwhile, place the apricot slivers in a large bowl. Then, in a jug, combine half the spring onions, all the lemon juice, rind, olive oil and seasoning, and pour over the apricot slivers.

Place a large saucepan over medium heat, add the cumin and coriander and stir continuously for 1–2 minutes, until you can smell their aroma. Add the mushrooms and stir until they are coated with the spices, and then cook for about 15 minutes, until their juices are released and they become dry. Remove from the heat.

Meanwhile, add the baked onions to the apricot mixture.

Add the lentils to the mushrooms, and then mix them through the apricot mixture. (You want the lentils to maintain their shape and still be slightly warm when you eat them, so stir them in carefully.)

Sprinkle with the remaining spring onions, pine nuts and coriander or parsley, and serve immediately with slices of avocado and on a bed of fresh green leaves.

Variations

Replace the pine nuts with almonds, shelled pistachios or sunflower seeds.

If you cannot find dried apricots, use 5–6 fresh apricots instead.

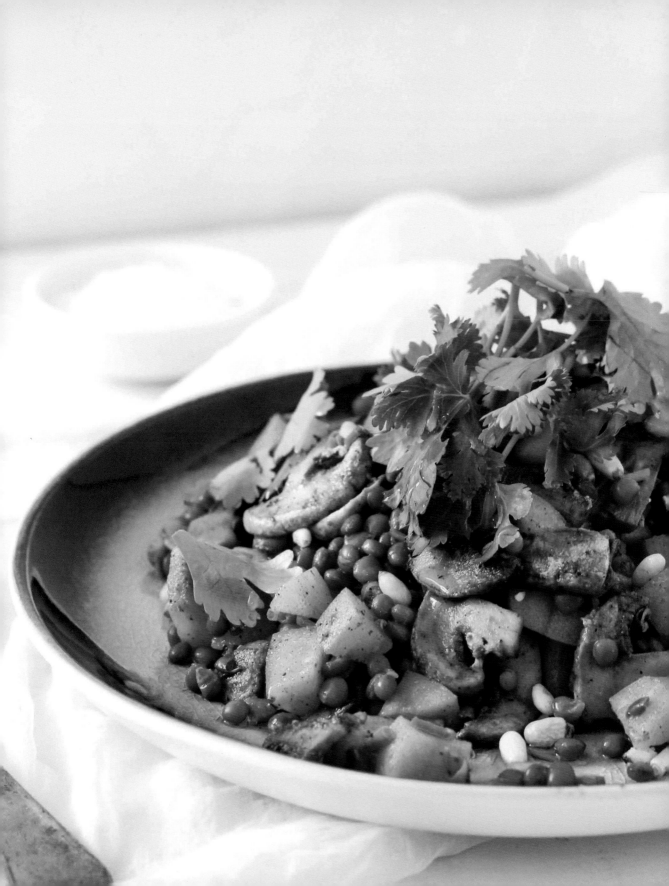

CHINESE GREENS AND BAKED TOFU SALAD

PREPARATION: 45 MINUTES | SERVES 6

This is a meal in itself. The greens add crunch and the tofu brings a delicious bite. Improvise with other Chinese greens if you can't find the exact ones in your supermarket.

½ Chinese cabbage, torn into bite-sized pieces

5 spring onions (shallots, scallions), thinly sliced

5 cups other Chinese greens, such as bok choy, sliced into strips

baked tofu (see below)

few sprigs fresh coriander (cilantro), to serve

Baked tofu

2 x 300-gram (10-ounce) blocks plain, hard (firm) organic tofu, cut into squares (each the size of a large dice)

Sauce

2 tablespoons gluten-free miso

2 tablespoons gluten-free soya (soy) sauce

3 garlic cloves

1 tablespoon grated ginger or a 3-centimetre/1-inch knob of ginger

1 tablespoon cumin

1 tablespoon ground coriander

3 tablespoons coconut milk

squeeze of lemon juice

Preheat the oven to 150°C/300°F. Line a baking tray with baking paper.

Spread the chopped tofu onto the baking paper.

Combine the sauce ingredients in a blender or food processor and blend until thick and creamy. Pour over the tofu and toss lightly until all the tofu is evenly covered with the sauce.

Place the marinated tofu in the oven and bake for 40 minutes, until the tofu is light golden in colour.

Remove from the oven and allow to cool slightly.

In a large bowl, combine all the Chinese greens, then add the slightly cooled tofu. Sprinkle the coriander over the salad. Serve with the pine nut mayonnaise (see recipe on page 69) or the roasted garlic (2) dressing (see recipe on page 71). Alternatively, I have used the peanut satay sauce (see recipe on page 78), diluted with a little coconut milk, as a great dressing too.

Tip
You can use this tofu for the above salad or make extra and refrigerate in an airtight glass container for a couple of days and toss into other salads for extra protein and flavour. Try to marinate the tofu the day before, so that the flavours develop well, but if you can't, it's still delicious. Remember to use hard (firm) tofu. The silken tofu will fall apart, and the recipe won't work.

SPICY MEXICAN BEAN SALAD

PREPARATION: 20 MINUTES | SERVES 4–6

In this recipe the spices work beautifully with the beans, tomatoes and red capsicum (bell pepper) to produce a very tasty, high-protein salad that you can serve with fresh tortillas and avocado salsa (see recipe on page 81) or plain mashed avocado with a squeeze of lemon juice and a sprinkle of salt. Serve it on a bed of baby spinach leaves or rocket (arugula) for added nutrients and greens. You can also serve it on baked corn 'chips' topped with avocado salsa topped with a dollop of savoury cashew cream (see options on page 32) and some lemon or lime wedges.

Salad

1⅓ cup cooked borlotti beans or 1 can (425 grams/ 15 ounces), drained

1⅓ cups cooked cannellini beans or 1 can (425 grams/ 15 ounces), drained

½ cup sun-dried tomatoes, finely sliced

¼ small red onion, peeled and finely chopped

1 medium red capsicum (bell pepper), chopped into cubes

10 baby tomatoes, halved

1 small bunch fresh coriander (cilantro), chopped

Dressing

¼ cup soaked and drained cashew nuts

juice of 1 small lemon or lime

¼ teaspoon ground cumin

¼ teaspoon ground coriander

½ teaspoon paprika

1 garlic clove, peeled

¼ cup water

salt and pepper, to taste

To make the salad, combine all the ingredients in a large glass bowl.

To make the dressing, combine all the ingredients in a blender and blend until smooth and creamy. Pour over the salad to serve.

Variations

Replace the red onion with 5–6 spring onions (shallots, scallions), green stalks included.

Replace the cashew nuts with macadamia nuts.

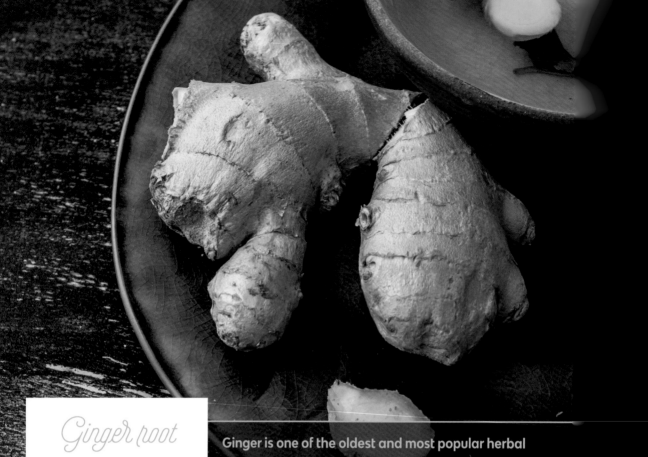

Ginger root

Ginger is one of the oldest and most popular herbal medicines. This rhizome, originally from the tropical jungles of South-East Asia, was one of the first exotic spices to reach the West, travelling along the spice route to the Mediterranean and England, where it was an important ingredient for making gingerbread in medieval times. The fresh root of ginger is an antioxidant and has also been shown to be helpful in lowering triglyceride levels. Some research suggests that ginger may be useful in delaying the onset and progression of cognitive decline, probably due to its ability to act as a circulatory stimulant. There has been some concern that it may have the potential to thin your blood, especially if you are on other pharmaceutical blood-thinners. Ginger tea is made easily by steeping a few fresh root ginger slices in hot water for a few minutes. This tea may calm and soothe the stomach after digestive challenges, as well as prevent colds and flu. Recent research has confirmed that ginger is successful at preventing nausea and may be more effective than prescribed drugs — whether for travel sickness, anxiety, pregnancy, over-eating or a stomach bug.

SOUPS

Soups can be delicious and soothing and are often associated with emotionally comforting childhood memories. They are also often served to people who are feeling ill or recovering from a physical ailment. However, soups can also easily form the backbone of a main meal when served with a lovely large salad.

Bean and root-vegetable soups can cook for ages, while soups that contain delicate vegetables, such as broccoli, are best served with minimal cooking. I've combined these approaches so that you still retain most of the nutrients — and colour — from vegetables that don't need to cook for a long period.

Most vegetable stock contains hydrolyzed vegetable protein (HVP), which is just another name for monosodium glutamate (MSG). MSG is toxic to brain cells in the concentrations found in these products and should be avoided, so I only use a non-HVP product.

Garnishing soups can be a fun way to add more nutrients in a visibly appealing way. Use herbs of contrasting colour and some finely chopped fresh vegetable to add crunch appeal and increase nutritional value. Herb oils (see page 84) along with fresh herbs can really enhance the flavour of soup — try tarragon with mushrooms, basil with tomato-based soups, and chopped coriander (cilantro) with corn-based soups. Spices add depth and character — use a pinch of nutmeg with mushroom soups, and curry powder with sweet potato, pumpkin (winter squash) or cauliflower soups. Freshly grated ginger adds special flavour to soups with pumpkin or carrots — add it just before serving for the freshest taste.

GLUTEN-FREE FLAT BREAD

PREPARATION: 15 MINUTES (PLUS 20–25 MINUTES BAKING TIME) | SERVES 6–8

Most people who give up gluten miss bread the most, and it's very challenging to make a gluten-free bread that competes with a gluten one. For this reason I haven't tried to do so and have instead made a high-protein flat bread that is great to serve with avocado salsa (see recipe on page 81) and soups. The trick is to eat it while it is still warm from the oven, so prepare all your other dishes and then pop it into the oven so that you can eat it when it is done. Break it into chunks to enjoy.

½ cup chickpea (besan, gram) flour

½ cup gluten-free 1 flour (see recipe on page 33)

½ cup polenta

1 teaspoon dried Italian herbs

1 teaspoon herb salt

1½ cups water

1 teaspoon psyllium husks

1¼ teaspoons baking powder

few sprigs of fresh rosemary

1 small onion, peeled and thickly sliced

Preheat the oven to 190°C/375°C. Prepare a baking tray (20 x 25 centimetres/8 x 10 inches).

In a bowl, combine the flours, polenta, herbs, herb salt, water and psyllium husks. Set aside for 15 minutes.

Add the baking powder, stirring to combine, and then pour into the baking tray, spreading the mixture evenly. Layer the rosemary sprigs and onion slices on the top, and bake for 15–20 minutes, until the flat bread comes away from the sides of the baking tray. Sprinkle a little olive oil over the bread and serve immediately.

CREAMY SWEET POTATO AND GINGER SOUP

PREPARATION: 40 MINUTES | SERVES 4–6

After tasting something similar in a restaurant, I decided to experiment in my kitchen but without the added milk, cream, butter and chicken stock. The result is a warming and refreshing soup, with just a hint of heat from the fresh ginger. I like to top this soup with the coriander (cilantro) herb oil (see recipe on page 84) and some grated orange rind, but a few sprigs of coriander (cilantro) work well too.

1 large onion, peeled and finely chopped

2 garlic cloves, peeled and crushed

2 tablespoons chopped fresh ginger

2 heaped teaspoons mild curry powder (see recipe on page 85)

1 can (400 millilitres/13 fluid ounces) coconut cream

3 medium sweet potatoes, roughly chopped

3 medium carrots, roughly chopped

4 cups vegetable stock

juice and rind of 1 large orange

salt and pepper, to taste

coriander (cilantro) or finely sliced ginger, to garnish

In a large saucepan, combine the onion, garlic, ginger and curry powder. Pour in a few tablespoons of the coconut cream and place over medium heat for 2 minutes to lightly sauté. Add the sweet potato, carrot, stock, juice and rind (keeping a few strands for serving) and simmer for 20–30 minutes until the vegetables are soft.

Remove from the heat and transfer the mixture to a blender or food processor. Blend until smooth, then return the mixture to the heat and stir in the remaining coconut milk and season to taste.

Serve at once, topping with coriander (cilantro) oil (see recipe on page 84), or coriander (cilantro) sprigs and remaining orange rind.

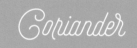

Coriander (cilantro) was one of the first herbs ever used in cooking and is mentioned in Sanskrit texts dating back 7000 years. The fresh leaves are rich in beta-carotene, which converts to vitamin A and vitamin C, both antioxidants, as well as vitamin B3 and the minerals iron and calcium. There is research to support the possible role of coriander in helping to remove heavy metals from the body, which may be very useful, because heavy metals pose a dangerous threat to delicate brain cells.

QUICK BEAN SOUP

PREPARATION: 1 HOUR | SERVES 4

This is so simple — if you have these ingredients in your pantry, you merely throw them all together and you have a tasty soup in an hour. Served with the gluten-free flat bread (see recipe on page 120) and a large leafy salad (see pages 89–117) you will have a very satisfying meal. The variation below, using lentils instead of the beans, is my son's favourite soup of all time and I could make it in my sleep by now.

2⅔ cups cooked beans of any variety or 2 cans (425 grams/15 ounces) borlotti or cannellini beans, drained

1 large carrot, finely chopped, or julienned

1 medium sweet potato, roughly grated

2 medium onions, peeled and roughly chopped

1 celery stick, finely chopped, including the leaves

2 large garlic cloves, sliced

1 tablespoon dried Italian herbs

1 bottle (500 grams/17½ ounces) pasta sauce, or ¼ cup tomato paste

3 cups water

few sprigs fresh basil

In a medium-sized saucepan combine all the ingredients except the basil. Place over a low heat and simmer for about an hour. Remove from the heat and use a potato masher to crush some of the vegetables and beans until you have crushed about half of the mixture, which provides a lovely balance of textures.

Serve topped with the fresh basil, green pesto (see recipe on page 73) or basil herb oil (see recipe on page 84).

Variations

Use lentils or chickpeas (garbanzo beans) instead of the beans.

Add 1 tablespoon of red pepper flakes to add a little heat.

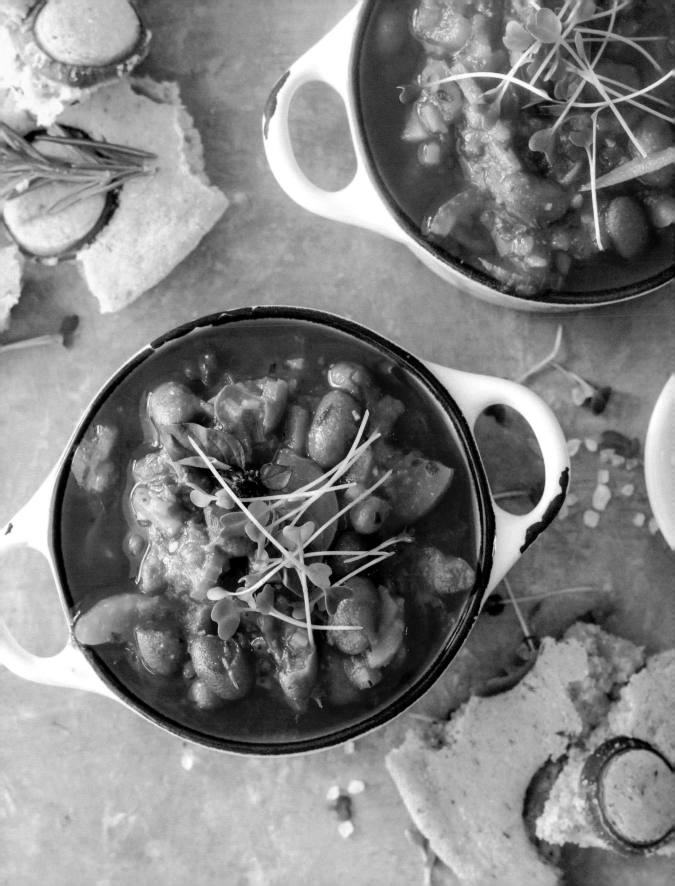

LENTIL DAHL

PREPARATION: 45–60 MINUTES | SERVES 6

Being able to quickly throw together the ingredients for this dish is very useful when you need to make something that can look after itself once it is assembled. As long as you've soaked the lentils, you can quickly get the rest of the ingredients together. If you don't have any sticks simply add fresh, finely ground cinnamon. I like to soak double the amount of lentils that the recipe calls for, then freeze half of them after draining them so that next time I make the dish, I don't have to do any soaking. You can use either yellow Chana dahl lentils, which take longer to cook, or red split lentils, which take less time. Either way this is a great, satisfying, nourishing meal.

4 tablespoons coconut oil

1 tablespoon black mustard seeds

1 tablespoon medium curry powder (see recipe on page 85)

1 heaped teaspoon turmeric powder

15 fresh curry leaves, finely chopped or left whole

2 medium red onions, peeled and thinly sliced

1 large carrot, finely chopped or grated

3 large garlic cloves, peeled and thinly sliced

1 teaspoon grated ginger

1½ cups yellow Chana dahl lentils or red split lentils, picked through to make sure there are no stones, then soaked for a whole day or night and then drained well

1 can (400 millilitres/13 fluid ounces) coconut cream, leaving a few teaspoons in the can to serve

3 cups boiling water

2 cinnamon sticks or ½ teaspoon finely ground fresh cinnamon

herb salt, to taste

½ bunch fresh coriander (cilantro), finely chopped

Add the coconut oil to a large saucepan and place over high heat. When the oil is hot, add the mustard seeds and place a lid on the saucepan. Wait for the sound of popping, about 30 seconds, then immediately remove from the heat, shake the saucepan to distribute the heat and wait until the popping subsides, which will take 2–3 minutes.

Return the saucepan to the heat. Remove the lid and add the curry powder, turmeric and curry leaves. Stir to combine, then add the onions, carrot, garlic and ginger, stirring again.

Add the drained lentils and stir to coat with the spices, then add the coconut cream (retaining a little to drizzle over before serving) and water. Bring the mixture to the boil, then add the two whole cinnamon sticks and allow them to cook with the lentils.

Reduce the heat to a simmer and continue to cook until the lentils are completely soft. The time will depend on whether you are using the harder and bigger yellow Chana dahl lentils or the smaller, softer split red lentils. It will take anywhere from 40–90 minutes for the yellow lentils and about 30–40 minutes for the red lentils.

Add the herb salt to taste, stir, and turn the heat off.

Serve with a good sprinkle of chopped coriander and the remaining drizzle of coconut cream. If you have prepared it for the next day, don't add the coriander until serving.

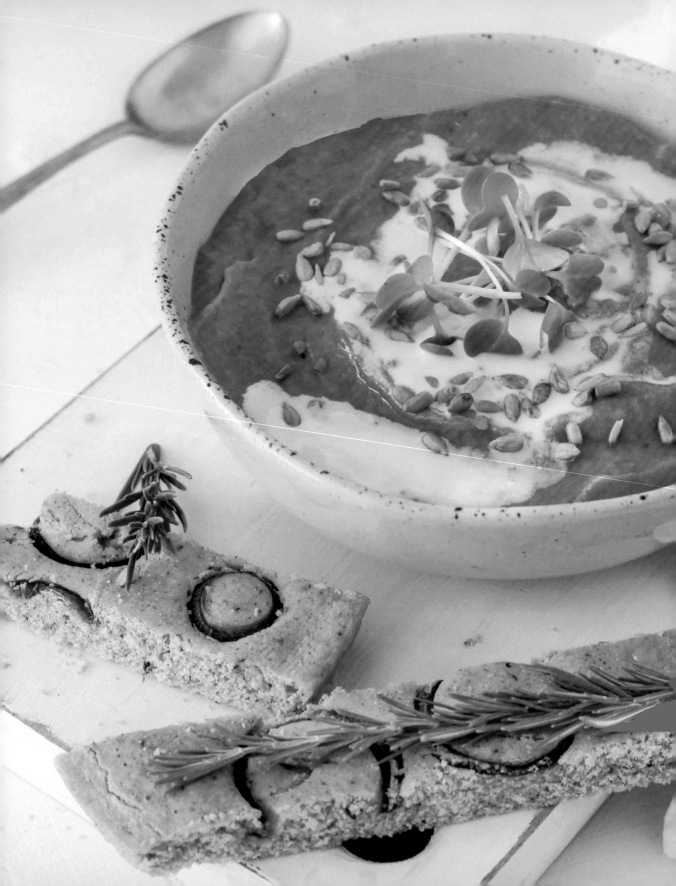

MAGICAL CREAMED SOUP BASE

PREPARATION: 40 MINUTES | SERVES 4–6

With this base you simply add a variety of vegetables and get a new soup each time. It's easy to make, and nutritious, because your vegetable of choice doesn't cook until it is mushy, and the colours stay appealing. We don't add the cashew nut cream or coconut milk every time we make one of these soups, because the potato makes the soup quite creamy as it is. A sprinkle of nuts or seeds as well as herbs adds extra crunch and nutrition to any of these variations.

3 medium potatoes, roughly chopped

1 medium onion, peeled and sliced

1 garlic clove, peeled

3 cups vegetable stock

½ cup coconut cream (optional)

2–3 tablespoons olive oil (optional)

½ cup savoury cashew nut cream (see options on page 32 — use a third of the quantities and use the leftovers to make a mayonnaise) (optional)

salt, to taste

2–3 cups vegetable of choice (see variations)

Add the potatoes, onion, garlic and stock to a large saucepan and place over a low heat to simmer for 25 minutes, until cooked.

Meanwhile, lightly steam your choice of vegetable, then add to the potato base. With a hand-held electric blender, blend the mixture until smooth. Remove from the heat and add the coconut cream, some olive oil or some cashew nut cream.

To garnish, use any fresh herb of choice — coriander, basil, chives, thyme or even cinnamon for butternut pumpkin (squash) soup.

Variations

Pumpkin (winter squash) soup: Use the above base and steam a medium pumpkin until soft, or bake it in the oven for about 45 minutes, at 150°C/300°F, remembering to prick it all over with a sharp knife before baking. Sauté 1 medium onion and 2 crushed garlic cloves with 1 tablespoon mild curry powder (see recipe on page 85) in a few tablespoons of coconut cream until the onions soften, which will take about 5 minutes. Blend the base ingredients, pumpkin and 1 can (400 millilitres/13 fluid ounces) coconut cream. Reheat but do not boil. Serve immediately with a sprinkle of coriander (cilantro) leaves or coriander (cilantro) oil (see page 84).

Broccoli soup: Use the above base and add 1 medium lightly steamed broccoli. Blend well. You can add ½ cup cashew nut cream (see options on page 32) with 2 tablespoons fresh lemon juice to give it a really creamy, fresh flavour. Reheat but do not boil. Serve immediately with a sprinkle of fresh or smoked paprika, or some finely chopped red capsicum (bell pepper) — or some finely chopped chillies (chili peppers) if you want some heat. You could add a drizzle of any of the herb oils (see page 84) or a dollop of instant sun-dried tomato pesto (see the tip on page 73).

Sweet potato soup: Use the above base and add 1 roughly chopped sweet potato, and blend well with the same curry and onion blend that the pumpkin soup above uses.

Cauliflower soup: Use the above base and add 1 medium cauliflower 10 minutes before the potatoes are done. Blend well and use the same curry and onion blend that the pumpkin soup uses, adding a tiny pinch of fresh nutmeg to the mixture too, or drizzle one of the herb or red capsicum (bell pepper) oils (see page 84) over the soup before serving.

Carrot soup: Use the above base and add 2 chopped medium carrots 15 minutes before the potatoes are done. Blend well and add 1 cup cashew nut cream (see options on page 32) with 2 tablespoons fresh lemon juice. Reheat but do not boil. Serve immediately with chopped chives and red pepper flakes, or coriander (cilantro) oil (see page 84), as garnish.

Roasted red capsicum (bell pepper) soup: Use the above base and roast 3 medium red capsicum (bell peppers) (see page 71). Lightly sauté 1 teaspoon each of cumin, coriander and paprika in a few tablespoons of coconut cream. Add 2 cups fresh cabbage 10 minutes before the potatoes are done. Blend these ingredients with the skinned and de-seeded roasted capsicum, 1 can (400 millilitres/13 fluid ounces) coconut milk and ⅓ cup tomato paste until smooth. Reheat but do not boil. Serve immediately with fresh basil leaves as garnish, a sprinkling of paprika and a swirl of coconut milk. The basil oil (see recipe on page 84) is excellent with this soup.

Sweet corn chowder: Use the above base and lightly steam 2 cups sweet corn, either from frozen or cut off the cob. Blend the base ingredients and the sweet corn roughly, so there are still chunks of vegetables, and return to the stove to reheat, but do not boil. Serve immediately with finely chopped sun-dried tomatoes and some finely chopped red capsicum (bell pepper) or red capsicum oil (see recipe on page 84). Finely chopped chives also look good — the bright colours are lovely and the soup is a very tasty alternative to the milk-and-cream-laden version. If the mixture is a little too thick, simply add ½–1 cup rice milk to thin it down.

PUMPKIN (WINTER SQUASH) AND LEMONGRASS SOUP WITH GREMOLATA

PREPARATION: 45 MINUTES | SERVES 6–8

This is a refreshing yet rich and smooth soup. The lemongrass adds a citrusy, exotic flavour, while the coconut milk brings depth and richness. Don't leave the gremolata out — it rounds the soup off wonderfully. It is a little more time-consuming than the other soups in this book, so make it for guests the day before, and simply heat lightly just before serving. Serving this soup cold is just as delicious, and very convenient! If you don't like a strong lemon flavour, and would prefer the coconut flavour to dominate, then just add 1 tablespoon (rather than 4) of the lemon juice at the end of cooking. When you serve the soup cold, all 4 tablespoons make it very light and citrusy. It saves a lot of time if you bake the pumpkin first.

Soup
- 1 medium–large pumpkin (winter squash)
- 4 cups vegetable stock
- 1 large onion, peeled and roughly chopped
- 1 x 5-centimetre/2-inch knob ginger, finely sliced
- 10 fresh coriander (cilantro) stems, washed well and leaves saved for gremolata, below
- 2 sticks lemongrass
- 1 can (400 millilitres/13 fluid ounces) coconut milk
- juice of 2 lemons (set aside the zest for the gremolata, below, before you squeeze the juice)
- salt and pepper, to taste

Gremolata
- 1 tablespoon sesame oil or olive oil
- zest of 2 lemons, finely chopped
- 1 teaspoon minced garlic
- ¼ cup chopped fresh coriander (cilantro)

Preheat the oven to 150°C/300°F. Line a baking tray with baking paper.

With a large, sharp knife, prick the pumpkin skin evenly, about 20 times, and place on the baking tray. Bake for 45–60 minutes, until soft. Remove from the oven and scoop out the flesh, discarding the seeds.

Meanwhile, combine the stock, onion, ginger, coriander stems and lemongrass in a large saucepan. Place over high heat and bring to the boil, then reduce heat, cover and simmer for 15–20 minutes, until the onion and lemongrass are soft.

Remove the lemongrass and coriander stems, and then transfer the mixture to a blender or food processor. Add the pumpkin in batches, blending each time until smooth.

Return the mixture to the saucepan and stir in the coconut milk (leaving a few teaspoons to use as garnish), lemon juice and salt and pepper to taste. Turn on the heat but do not boil the soup — heat it only to serving temperature.

While the soup is simmering, make the gremolata, combining all the ingredients in a small bowl.

Garnish the soup in bowls with 1 teaspoon of gremolata.

CREAM OF MUSHROOM SOUP

PREPARATION: 30 MINUTES (PLUS SOAKING TIME) | SERVES 4–6

Mushroom soup is very satisfying soup on a cold wintery day. Mushrooms impart a woody, robust flavour to most dishes, and this soup is no exception. You can leave out the cashew nut cream, because the potatoes do give the soup a creamy texture, but I find the addition of the nut cream adds extra creaminess.

1 cup dried porcini mushrooms

½ cup water

2 medium potatoes, chopped

1 large onion, peeled and finely chopped

1 garlic clove, peeled and crushed

2 cups plain vegetable stock

1 punnet (or 2 cups) large brown mushrooms, chopped

1 punnet (or 2 cups) white button mushrooms, chopped

salt and pepper, to taste

1 cup cashew nut cream (see options on page 32)

2 tablespoons finely diced fresh thyme or fresh nutmeg, to garnish

Wash the porcini very well under running water to get rid of any small pieces of sand or twigs. Place them in a bowl and cover them with ½ cup water, then let them stand for 2 hours.

Remove the porcini from the soaking liquid (but retain this liquid) and rinse them well. Chop them and set aside. Pour the porcini soaking liquid through a very fine sieve (or clean coffee filter) to catch any sand or twigs, and set aside.

Meanwhile, place the potatoes, onion and garlic in a saucepan and pour over the stock. Place over medium heat and cook for 20 minutes, until just tender.

Add the porcini to the potato mixture along with the other mushrooms, then pour in the cleaned porcini soaking liquid. Stir and return to a simmer for 15 minutes, until the porcini are tender.

Remove from the heat and use a hand-held electric blender to blend the mixture until smooth, but leave a few chunky mushroom pieces. Season to taste with salt and pepper.

Add the cashew nut cream, reserving a few tablespoons for serving, and serve immediately with a splash of cashew nut cream and a sprinkling of fresh thyme or nutmeg.

Mushrooms

The ancient Egyptians decreed mushrooms only fit for royalty, while other civilizations throughout Europe, Russia, China, Mexico and Latin America practised mushroom rituals. France was the leader in the formal cultivation of edible mushrooms. Mushrooms are not a vegetable, but belong to the fungi family. They contain potassium, iron, selenium and zinc, as well as vitamins B1, B2, B3, B5 and D. Porcini mushrooms contain anti-inflammatory compounds, along with a compound called ergosterol, which attacks invading bacteria or viruses. In animal studies, Maitake mushrooms have been shown to protect against cardiovascular disease and cancer, and lower blood pressure and regulate blood glucose, both activities that protect the brain. Shiitake mushrooms contain potent anti-cancer agents, and Reishi mushrooms are very high in antioxidant activity, containing a phytonutrient called ganoderic acid.

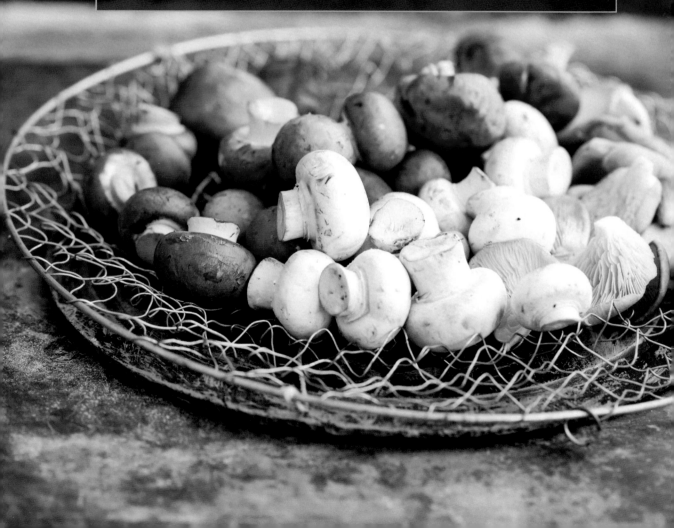

Onions

Onions have been cultivated for 6000 years — without any botanist discovering a variety that doesn't produce tears! They are believed to have originated in the Middle East, and it is likely they spread quickly due to their easy cultivation. Onions contain some B vitamins, vitamin C and K and as well as calcium, iron, manganese, magnesium, copper and potassium. They also contain a wide variety of flavonoids, which improve health by lowering bad cholesterol and reducing the risk of heart disease. They also have antibacterial and antiviral properties, and contain quercetin, a powerful antioxidant. The red onion is the best choice as a brain food, simply due to its antioxidant pigment, and spring onions (shallots, scallions) are also nutritious, especially if you also use their green stems.

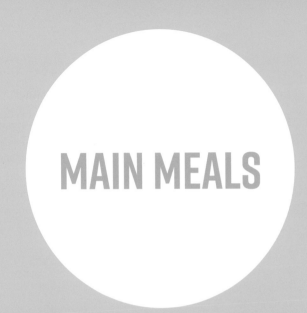

MAIN MEALS

Main meals that leave you feeling too full and tired are not a great idea, but these plant-based main meals won't do that. When you are used to eating large meals it may come as a shock to discover that you don't need to eat vast quantities of food to feel satisfied. And over time, you will find yourself preferring to eat smaller main meals, and have more vegetables in the form of salads, as side dishes. The aim of food is to satisfy our taste buds and provide us with nutrients. These mains are delicious, nutrient dense, prepared with health in mind and have many variations that you can play with.

There are no animal products in these recipes due to the likely presence of hormones, pesticides and heavy metals that accumulate in them, which are particularly harmful to our health, especially our sensitive brain. In addition, most animals are grain fed, which means they contain too much omega-6 and very little omega-3 essential fatty acids.

Curries are one of the tastiest ways to enjoy vegetables, and I prefer to make curries that children can also enjoy, so I don't add chillies, instead focusing on the spiciness of the dish. However, if you want to add chillies (chili peppers), please do. Making your own curry pastes — if you have the time — ensures that you are using the freshest ingredients possible. There are, however, some good pastes available now; just be sure to check for the absence of unnecessary preservatives, colourants and flavourings.

Some of these recipes are time consuming, so are best prepared when you have some extra time, although being well organized and prepared will make their preparation simple. I find that I generally serve larger main meals on the weekend when I entertain and have a little extra time to spend in my kitchen.

SLOW-BAKED SWEET POTATO, PUMPKIN (SQUASH) AND COCONUT CURRY

PREPARATION: 60 MINUTES (PLUS 2 HOURS BAKING TIME) | SERVES 8–10

This curry is baked in the oven and is useful when you are expecting guests, because it can be prepared the day before, refrigerated, and then just popped into the oven a couple of hours before eating. By starting the meal with a large, fresh, raw salad, you still get in plenty of fresh vegetables. Cooking this curry slowly ensures that the flavours are intense. As it is more spicy than hot, even children enjoy it — however, if you want it more potent, simply use about 4 tablespoons of curry powder instead of the 2. Visiting the Seychelles taught me that cinnamon elevates a curry from good to sublime!

1⅓ cups cooked lentils (reserving water) or 1 can (425 grams/15 ounces), undrained

1½ cans (400 millilitres/13 fluid ounces, plus 200 millilitres/7 fluid ounces) coconut cream

1 teaspoon mustard seeds

2 teaspoons cinnamon

1 tablespoon grated ginger or 8-centimetre/3-inch knob of ginger

2 tablespoons mild curry powder (see recipe on page 85)

6 garlic cloves, peeled and crushed

3 large onions, peeled and finely sliced

3 small sweet potatoes, peeled and chopped into cubes

½ medium butternut pumpkin (squash), peeled and chopped into cubes

1 bunch or ½ cup fresh coriander (cilantro), finely chopped

juice and rind of 2 oranges

salt and pepper, to taste

Preheat the oven to 160°C/320°F.

Set aside the lentils' soaking liquid.

In a saucepan, combine the coconut cream, mustard seeds, cinnamon, ginger, curry powder, garlic and onion. Place over medium heat for 5 minutes, until the aroma is released and the onions and garlic have sweated, then remove from the heat.

In a bowl, combine the sweet potatoes, pumpkin and lentils. Spread ⅓ of this mixture over the bottom of an ovenproof dish (with a lid), then cover this with half of the spicy mixture and top with a little salt, fresh coriander and orange rind. Repeat with the second third of the vegetable mixture and top with the remaining half of the spicy mixture, and top with a little salt and fresh coriander and orange rind. Finally, spread the final third of the sweet potato mixture on top, and sprinkle with a little salt, fresh coriander and orange rind.

In a jug, combine the rest of the coconut cream, orange juice and the leftover lentil water, and pour this mixture over everything when you have made all the layers.

Place the lid on the dish and bake, covered, for 90 minutes and then uncovered for 30 more minutes.

Serve with a combination of quinoa and millet, or brown basmati rice.

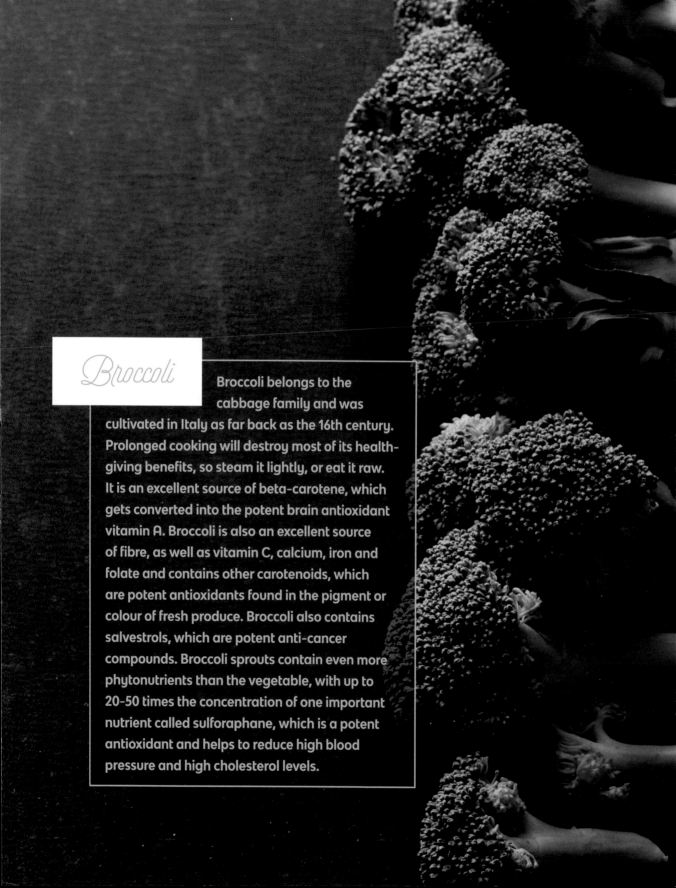

Broccoli

Broccoli belongs to the cabbage family and was cultivated in Italy as far back as the 16th century. Prolonged cooking will destroy most of its health-giving benefits, so steam it lightly, or eat it raw. It is an excellent source of beta-carotene, which gets converted into the potent brain antioxidant vitamin A. Broccoli is also an excellent source of fibre, as well as vitamin C, calcium, iron and folate and contains other carotenoids, which are potent antioxidants found in the pigment or colour of fresh produce. Broccoli also contains salvestrols, which are potent anti-cancer compounds. Broccoli sprouts contain even more phytonutrients than the vegetable, with up to 20-50 times the concentration of one important nutrient called sulforaphane, which is a potent antioxidant and helps to reduce high blood pressure and high cholesterol levels.

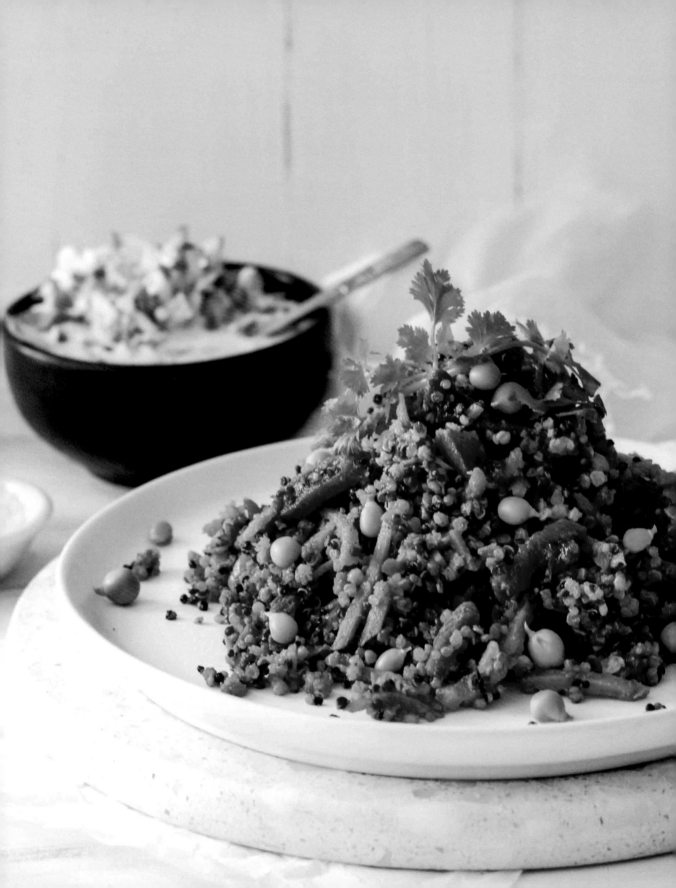

CURRIED CARROT, CHICKPEA (GARBANZO BEAN) AND QUINOA PILAF

PREPARATION: 30 MINUTES | SERVES 6

We were sailing in the Mediterranean and didn't have much fresh food left in our pantry, so we ended up combining chickpeas (garbanzo beans), apricots and curry to make a high-protein, colourful 'meal in a pot', which was very satisfying served with a large green salad. Don't be put off by the number of ingredients — it is very quick to assemble and cooks quickly too. Be sure to follow the time limits, because otherwise the quinoa may turn mushy. And you can use either chickpeas or lentils, or even green peas that you've steamed briefly, and stir in just before serving. I like using peas, because they are such a great bright green colour, which contrasts perfectly with the carrots. The curry powder and fresh coriander (cilantro) are must-haves, though! This dish always brings back memories of that wonderful trip!

2 tablespoons coconut oil

1 medium onion, peeled and finely sliced

1 large garlic clove, peeled and finely sliced

2 cups grated or julienned carrots

1 tablespoons curry powder (see recipe on page 85)

½ tablespoon turmeric

1 cup quinoa, rinsed and drained well

1¾ cups water, plus an extra 2 tablespoons

1 teaspoon herb salt

½ cup dried apricots, thinly sliced

1⅓ cups cooked chickpeas (garbanzo beans) or lentils, or 1 can (425 grams/15 ounces), drained, or about 1 cup lightly cooked green peas

1 small bunch coriander (cilantro), finely chopped

In a medium saucepan, heat the coconut oil slightly over a medium heat and add the onion, garlic, carrots, curry powder and turmeric, stirring to coat everything in the spices and oil, and allow the spices to heat slightly to release their aroma.

Add the quinoa and stir well, then add 1¾ cups water and herb salt and stir well again. Bring to the boil and cover with a tight-fitting lid, then reduce the heat to a simmer for 20 minutes.

Remove from the heat and lightly toss in the apricot slivers and legumes of choice, while fluffing the mixture up with two forks. Cover with the lid and set aside for about 10 minutes.

Add the coriander and serve with the cucumber cooler (see recipe on page 143) on the side and a large green salad with sliced avocado.

Variations

Replace the apricot slivers with ½ cup finely sliced preserved lemon or the rind of one fresh lemon or orange.

Replace the quinoa with brown basmati rice (which is what we did on our trip) and increase cooking time to 45 minutes.

Use either tri-coloured or plain white quinoa.

QUICK CHICKPEA (GARBANZO BEAN) AND SPINACH CURRY

PREPARATION: 15 MINUTES (PLUS 30 MINUTES COOKING TIME) | SERVES 4–6

When winter arrives I look forward to making this curry. It is rich and warming, with a lovely aroma. I serve it with quinoa, millet or brown basmati rice. A drizzle of coriander (cilantro) oil (see recipe on page 84) adds the final touch.

1 large onion, peeled and finely chopped

3 garlic cloves, peeled and crushed

1½ teaspoons finely grated ginger (8-centimetre/3-inch knob of ginger)

1 can (400 millilitres/13 fluid ounces) coconut cream

3 tablespoons mild curry powder (see recipe on page 85)

1 teaspoon turmeric

10 fresh curry leaves

1 small sweet potato, chopped into bite-sized pieces

½ medium butternut pumpkin (squash), chopped into bite-sized pieces

1 medium carrot, peeled and chopped into bite-sized pieces

1⅓ cups cooked chickpeas (garbanzo beans) or 1 can (425 grams/15 ounces), drained

2 cups baby spinach leaves, roughly chopped

small bunch coriander (cilantro), roughly chopped

salt and pepper, to taste

juice of 1 small lemon or lime

In a large saucepan, combine the onion, garlic and ginger with the coconut cream and cook over medium heat for a few minutes until the onion and garlic soften. Add the curry powder, turmeric and curry leaves and cook, stirring, for 5 minutes or until the aroma of the spices is released. Add the sweet potato, butternut pumpkin, carrot and chickpeas. Bring to the boil and then reduce the heat and simmer for about 30 minutes or until the vegetables are cooked, then turn off the heat.

Stir in the spinach and coriander, season to taste and stir in the lemon juice.

Serve immediately on your cooked grain of choice and garnish with coriander oil (see recipe on page 84) or green pesto (see recipe on page 73).

Variation
Serve with cucumber cooler (see recipe opposite).

Spinach

Spinach originated in Persia and by the end of the 1500s was popular in England, apparently due to Catherine de Medici's influence and the fact that it was a spring plant, available when other summer vegetables hadn't yet had a chance to mature. It is an excellent source of vitamin C if eaten raw, as well as vitamins A and B, and contains the minerals calcium, iron and potassium. Eat spinach with vitamin C-rich food because it contains oxalic acid, which inhibits the absorption of iron and calcium in the body.

CUCUMBER COOLER

PREPARATION: 10 MINUTES | MAKES 2 CUPS

This simple-to-prepare topping adds a refreshing flavour to most curries (see pages 134–42) along with extra nutrients.

1 large cucumber, sliced into matchsticks
½ cup coconut cream
juice of 1 large lemon
¼ cup fresh coriander (cilantro), finely chopped
¼ cup mint, finely chopped
2 spring onions (shallots, scallions), finely chopped
¼ cup desiccated coconut
salt, to taste

In a bowl, combine all the ingredients, and refrigerate until you are ready to serve.

Variation
Replace the coconut cream with the same amount of coconut yoghurt.

QUICK FRESH THAI STEW

PREPARATION: 30 MINUTES | SERVES 4–6

Once you've made the Thai spice paste (see recipe on page 86), this dish is simple to prepare, and has a lovely, fresh flavour.

1¼ cups coconut cream

1 medium onion, peeled and sliced

1 medium carrot, peeled and julienned into thick slices or sliced into half-circles

1 small sweet potato, chopped into bite-sized pieces

1 punnet (or 2 cups) button mushrooms, rinsed and halved (375 grams/ 13 ounces)

1 cup broccoli florets, chopped into bite-sized pieces

1 x 250 gram/9 ounce packet of buckwheat noodles

1 cup Thai spice paste (see recipe on page 86)

¼ cup finely sliced fresh coriander (cilantro)

¼ cup finely sliced spring onions (shallots, scallions)

Pour the coconut cream into a large saucepan and heat slowly over medium heat.

Add the onion, carrot, sweet potato and mushrooms, reduce heat and simmer for 15 minutes to cook the vegetables.

Meanwhile, cook the buckwheat noodles according to the packet instructions and drain well.

Add the broccoli to the vegetables in coconut cream and continue to simmer for 2–3 minutes, only until the broccoli is bright green and slightly tender.

Stir the Thai paste through the vegetables and stir in the well-drained noodles. Remove from the heat and divide between serving bowls, topping with the coriander and spring onions.

Variations

Toss in 1 cup of baked tofu (see recipe on page 116).

Replace the noodles with half a baked butternut pumpkin or squash (page 127) and scoop a few tablespoons of baked butternut into bowls, topped with the stew above, for each serve.

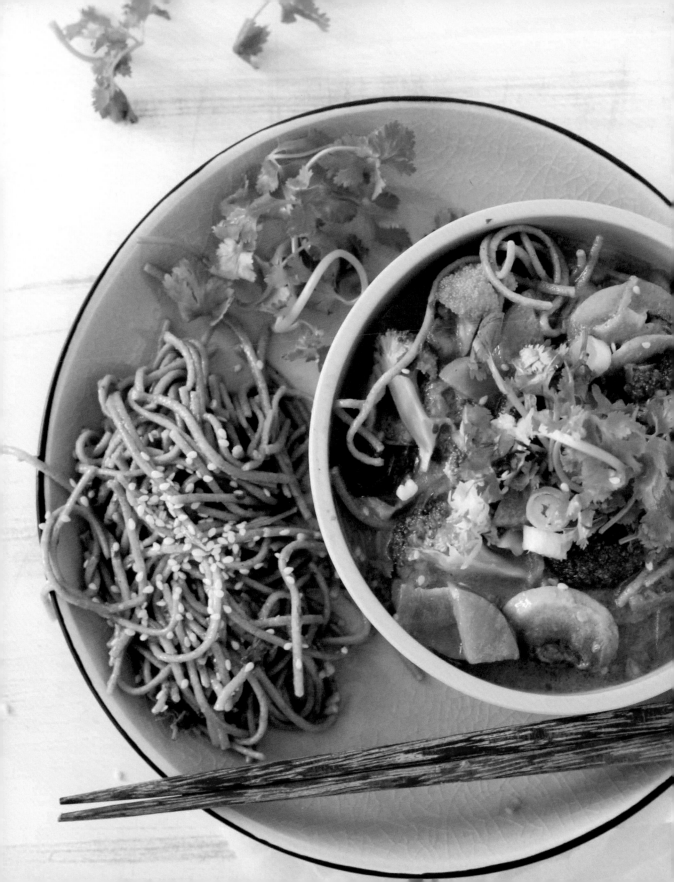

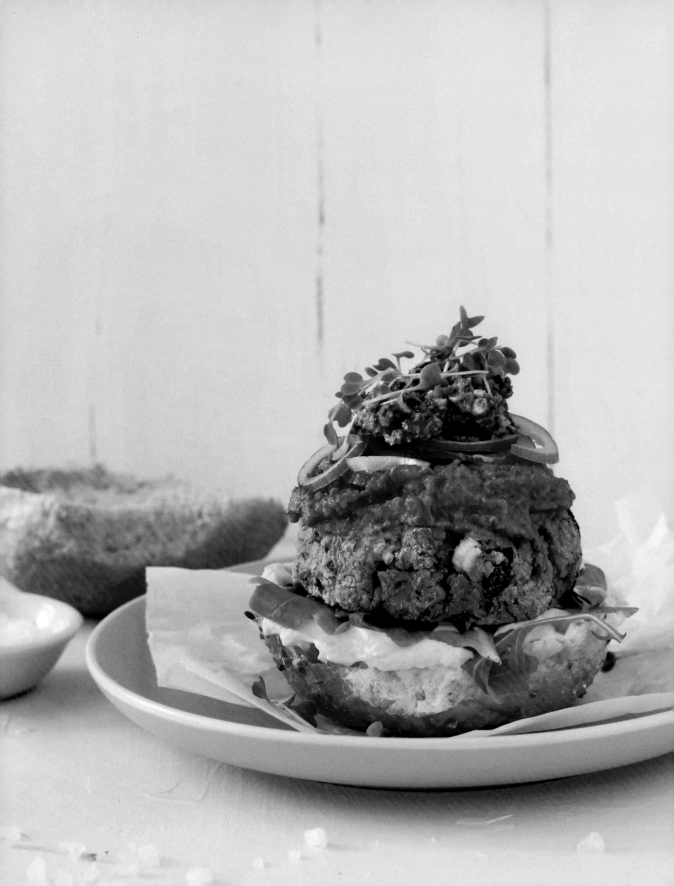

PECAN AND BEAN BURGERS

PREPARATION: 20 MINUTES | MAKES 8

These are very simple burgers to make and don't include any frying; the burgers are baked instead. The addition of pecans increases nutrient density and flavour, and topping them with a dollop of harissa sauce (see recipe on page 80), turmeric macadamia mayonnaise (see recipe on page 72) or green pesto (see recipe on page 73) adds to the lovely taste. I sometimes add a dollop of savoury cashew cream (see options on page 32) too. We use gluten-free bread or large baked mushrooms as a substitute for refined bread rolls, but these burgers are also delicious simply served with a green salad, such as that on page 96 or the golden coleslaw on page 92. If you don't have a food processor, simply grate the carrots and finely chop the onion and garlic and mash the beans with a potato masher. Serve with sweet potato 'chips' (page 175) for a healthy 'fast-food' meal.

2⅔ cups cooked chickpeas (garbanzo beans) or beans, or 2 cans (425 grams/ 15 ounces each), drained

1 large carrot, peeled and roughly chopped

1 medium onion, peeled and roughly chopped

1 garlic clove, peeled and finely sliced

⅓ cup pecans soaked in water for 2–3 hours, rinsed and drained well

3–4 spring onions (shallots, scallions), finely chopped

1 teaspoon dried thyme

1 teaspoon dried oregano (or Italian herbs)

handful of parsley or basil, finely chopped

1½ tablespoons psyllium husks

few tablespoons chickpea (besan, gram), tapioca or arrowroot flour, or quinoa flakes, for coating burgers

salt and pepper, to taste

Preheat the oven to 160°C/320°F. Line a baking tray with baking paper.

Combine the chickpeas or beans, carrot, onion, garlic and pecans in a food processor and pulse until they form a loose mixture with most of the ingredients in small chunks.

Transfer the mixture to a large bowl and toss in the spring onions, herbs and psyllium. Mix thoroughly.

Using a ½-cup measure, divide the mixture into equal quantities. Using your hands, shape them into flat patties, pressing down lightly and coating the patties in the flour or quinoa flakes.

Transfer the patties to the baking tray and bake for 30–40 minutes or until set. Serve with a variety of lettuce leaves, rocket (arugula), thinly sliced tomato, cucumber and red onions, and any of the variations above.

Variation
You can substitute lentils for the beans, but only add half the amount to the food processor and the other half after processing.

BAKED FALAFELS

PREPARATION: 15 MINUTES | MAKES 25

Falafels are delicious morsels of a spicy chickpea (garbanzo bean) mixture deep-fried — therefore they contain large quantities of damaged fat molecules. This is a healthier version, and sprinkling them with olive oil as you remove them from the oven provides the lovely oily mouthfeel without any toxic fat. Although I do not make a habit of rolling food into little balls I have made an exception for these tasty treats. They are best served with the tahini herb dressing from page 66 in a tortilla with fresh avocado salsa (see recipe on page 81) and a variety of green leaves. You can also use sturdy lettuce leaves in place of the tortillas. Although this makes for a very messy meal it's worth it! If you don't have a food processor, simply grate the carrots, finely chop the onion and parsley, and mash the chickpeas with a potato masher.

2⅔ cups cooked chickpeas (garbanzo beans), or 2 cans (425 grams/15 ounces each), drained

1 carrot, peeled and roughly chopped

½ red onion, peeled and roughly chopped

1 cup roughly chopped parsley

1 teaspoon ground cumin

1 teaspoon ground coriander

1 teaspoon herb salt

3 tablespoons either quinoa or amaranth flakes

1½ teaspoons psyllium husks

Preheat the oven to 160°C/320°F. Line a baking tray with baking paper.

Combine the chickpeas, carrot, onion, parsley, cumin and coriander in a food processor and pulse until you have a loose mixture with most of the ingredients in small chunks. Transfer the mixture to a bigger bowl and toss the herb salt, flakes and psyllium into the bowl and mix thoroughly.

Using a ⅛-cup measure (2 tablespoons), divide the mixture into equal quantities and using your hands, shape them into balls and place them on the baking tray. Bake for 45 minutes or until lightly golden in colour. Remove from the oven and drizzle olive oil over the balls and serve immediately.

Variations

Replace the chickpeas with cannellini beans.

Replace the parsley with fresh coriander (cilantro).

Replace the red onion with 3–4 finely chopped spring onions (shallots, scallions), green tips included.

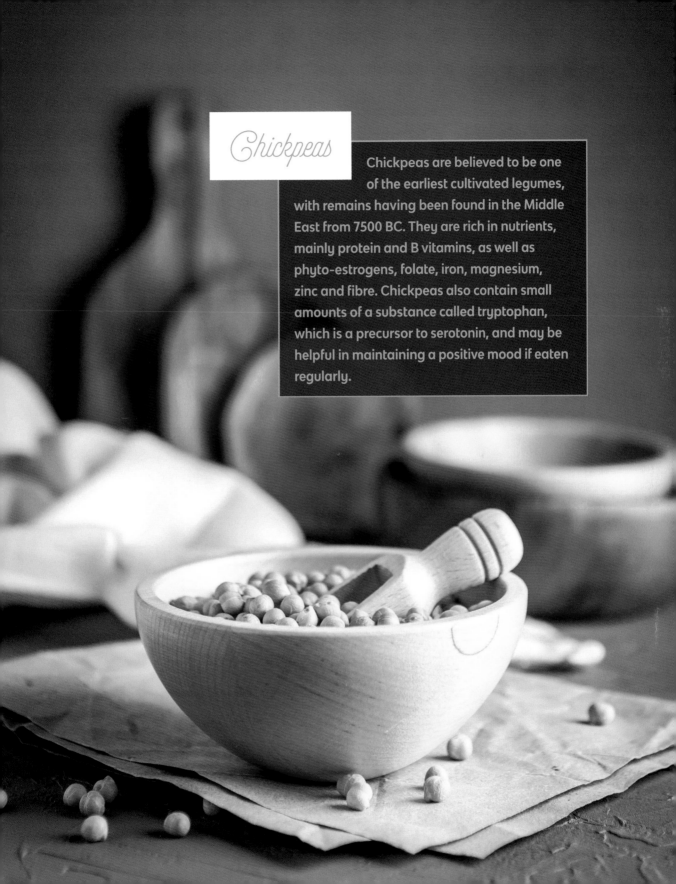

Chickpeas

Chickpeas are believed to be one of the earliest cultivated legumes, with remains having been found in the Middle East from 7500 BC. They are rich in nutrients, mainly protein and B vitamins, as well as phyto-estrogens, folate, iron, magnesium, zinc and fibre. Chickpeas also contain small amounts of a substance called tryptophan, which is a precursor to serotonin, and may be helpful in maintaining a positive mood if eaten regularly.

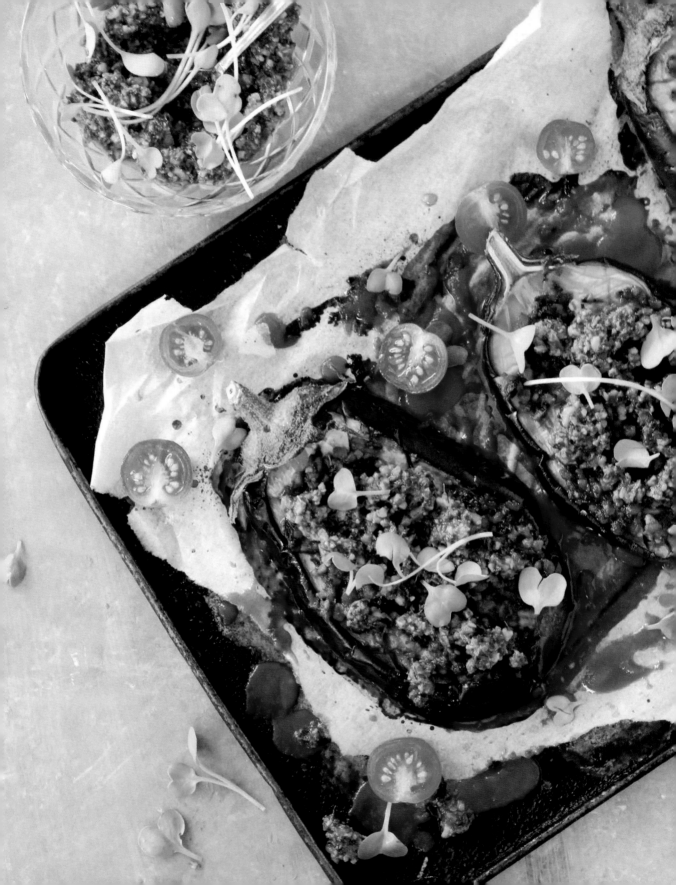

EGGPLANT (AUBERGINE) 'STEAKS'

PREPARATION: 1 HOUR | SERVES 6–8

This is not the quickest meal to prepare, but it is impressive when entertaining, because the flavours and textures are just so wonderful. The eggplants are reduced to buttery, melt-in-your mouth 'steaks' and both versions are simple to put together. Make this dish when you have time to allow the eggplants to marinate in either sauce for a few hours.

3 medium or 2 large
   eggplants (aubergine)

Slice the top and bottom from each eggplant, then slice horizontally into three thick slices or 'steaks' — 2.5 centimetres/1 inch thickness. Degorge if necessary (see tip on next page). Using a sharp knife, score on each side into even diamond shapes, deep enough to absorb the flavours while marinating, but not too deep to cut through the whole 'steak'.

Variation 1: Herb pesto steaks

1 cup green pesto (see recipe
   on page 73)

2 cups tomato sauce
   (see recipe on page 62),
   plus extra, to serve

salt and pepper, to taste

2–3 tablespoons fresh basil,
   finely chopped, to serve

Line a baking tray or large ovenproof baking dish with baking paper.

Divide the pesto between the eggplant slices, ensuring that you spread both sides of the 'steaks', and lay them on the baking tray or ovenproof dish. Top with equal quantities of the tomato sauce and set aside for a few hours to marinate.

Preheat the oven to 160°C/320°F.

Cover the baking tray with baking paper (or use the lid if you are using an ovenproof dish) and bake for 30 minutes. Reduce the heat to 110°C/230°F for the last 15 minutes until the 'steaks' are tender.

Serve with quinoa (see page 29).

Tip
You can replace the homemade tomato sauce with the same quantity of a good quality pasta sauce.

Variation 2: Curry steaks overleaf

Variation 2: Curry steaks

1 can (400 millilitres/13 fluid ounces) coconut milk

4 tablespoons mild curry paste or 4 tablespoons curry powder (see recipe on page 85)

2 large garlic cloves, peeled and crushed

salt and pepper, to taste

2–3 tablespoons coriander (cilantro), finely chopped, to serve

Line a baking tray or large ovenproof baking dish with baking paper.

In a bowl, combine half of the coconut milk (reserve the rest in an airtight container in the refrigerator) with the spices, garlic, salt and pepper, reserving the rest of the cream for cooking. Divide the spice mixture between the eggplant slices, ensuring that you coat both sides of the 'steaks' and lay them on the baking tray or ovenproof baking dish. Set aside for a few hours to marinate.

Preheat the oven to 160°C/320°F.

Pour the remaining coconut cream over the eggplant slices. Cover the baking tray with baking paper or use the lid if using an ovenproof dish, and bake for 30 minutes. Reduce the heat to 110°C/230°F for the last 15 minutes until the 'steaks' are tender.

Serve with quinoa (see page 29) tossed with ½ cup finely chopped fresh coriander and 1 tablespoon finely sliced fresh ginger, and 'Seychelles' tomato sauce (see recipe on page 62).

Tip

When eggplants are fresh their seeds are yellow and they are not bitter, so you don't have to degorge them. When the seeds are black or dark brown, then you must degorge them. Simply chop or slice them as per the recipe, and sprinkle salt over all the pieces. Put them in a colander so that the bitter juices can run out — this takes about an hour. Rinse them well before use.

SUPER-FAST PANTRY PASTA

PREPARATION: 20 MINUTES | SERVES 6

This pasta is one of our family's standby, super-fast meals. When dinner looms, and the day has been super-long and busy, I reach for a simple-to-make but nutritious meal. Sometimes I replace the green peas with chickpeas and the dish is just as tasty. Either way it is very satisfying and nutrient dense, and with a big dollop of pesto and avocado tossed through the pasta just before serving it's really satisfying.

250 grams/9 ounces (dried) gluten-free pasta

1 medium onion, peeled and finely sliced

2 bottles (2 x 250 grams/ 9 ounces each) or 1 can (425 grams/15 ounces) whole artichoke hearts, in water, drained

½ cup rice or almond milk

1 large garlic clove, peeled and finely sliced

3–4 tablespoons olive oil

75 grams capers, in salt, rinsed well, drained and roughly chopped

2 cups green peas, or 1⅓ cups cooked or 1 can (425 grams/15 ounces) chickpeas (garbanzo beans), drained and lightly crushed with a fork or potato masher

1 large avocado, peeled and chopped into small cubes

3–4 cups baby spinach, washed well and drained

1 cup green pesto (see recipe on page 73)

salt and pepper, to taste

few slices preserved lemon or the rind of 1 fresh lemon

Place a large saucepan of water over high heat and bring to the boil. Add the pasta to the boiling water, and when it reaches the halfway mark according to the packet instructions, usually about 4–5 minutes, add the onion. Allow the water to come back to the boil and start timing the pasta again from where you left off.

Meanwhile, combine the artichokes, rice or almond milk, garlic and olive oil in a blender or food processor and blend until smooth and creamy. Add the capers and pulse briefly to roughly chop them.

When the pasta is cooked, drain the water and return the pasta to the saucepan. Add the creamed artichoke mixture, chickpeas or peas, avocado, spinach leaves and pesto, and serve immediately topped with a sprinkle of preserved lemon.

The capers and preserved lemon contain salt, so you will probably not need to add any additional salt.

Variation

Replace the gluten-free pasta with the same amount of buckwheat noodles.

SWEET POTATO AND TOMATO GRATIN

PREPARATION: 15 MINUTES (PLUS 80 MINUTES BAKING TIME) | SERVES 4

To make a traditional gratin, white potatoes are layered in a dish with cream, milk or butter, topped with cheese and/or breadcrumbs and baked. In this dish I have used sweet potatoes, onion and garlic, along with coconut cream and store-bought pasta sauce, all of which is really simple to throw together, and it turns creamy and buttery when baked in this way. It's essential to use a mandolin, otherwise the slices will be too thick to get soft and creamy. Although it takes a long time to bake through, it is very simple to put together. Drizzling basil oil (see page 84) over this dish just before serving adds to the flavour and colour appeal, although I also love to add a dollop of lovely green pesto to my portion (see recipe on page 73). I serve this dish with a large salad that contains cooked legumes.

1 large sweet potato

1 large onion, peeled

1 cup coconut cream

5 garlic cloves, peeled and crushed

salt and pepper, to taste

1 cup tomato pasta sauce (see recipe on page 62)

¼ cup finely chopped fresh basil

Preheat the oven to 200°C/390°F. Prepare an 8–10 cup (2–2¼ quart) capacity ovenproof baking dish with a lid.

Use a mandolin to finely slice the potato and onion. In a bowl, combine the coconut cream, garlic, seasoning, tomato sauce and basil.

Spread a layer of potato and onion slices on the base of the baking dish.

Over the top, spread a layer of the coconut–tomato mixture. Continue this, alternating between a potato–onion layer and a coconut–tomato layer, until you have used all the mixtures — about three layers.

Place the lid on the baking dish and bake for 60 minutes. Reduce the temperature to 180°C/350°F and remove the lid for the last 15–20 minutes.

Slice into wedges and serve warm with a large leafy salad.

Variation
Add 2 tablespoons curry powder (see recipe on page 85) to the coconut mixture before blending. Replace the basil leaves with fresh coriander (cilantro).

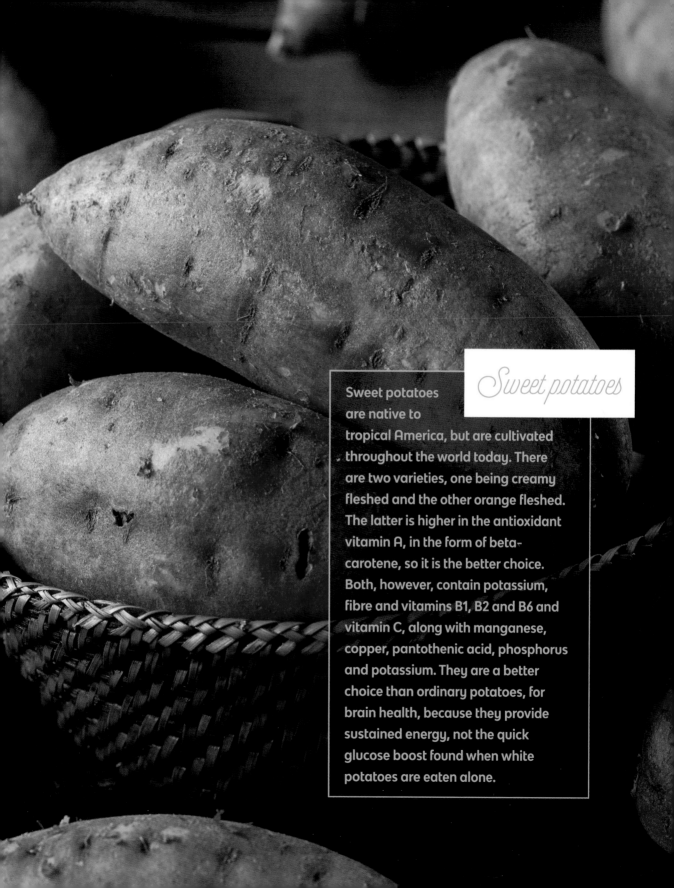

Sweet potatoes

Sweet potatoes are native to tropical America, but are cultivated throughout the world today. There are two varieties, one being creamy fleshed and the other orange fleshed. The latter is higher in the antioxidant vitamin A, in the form of beta-carotene, so it is the better choice. Both, however, contain potassium, fibre and vitamins B1, B2 and B6 and vitamin C, along with manganese, copper, pantothenic acid, phosphorus and potassium. They are a better choice than ordinary potatoes, for brain health, because they provide sustained energy, not the quick glucose boost found when white potatoes are eaten alone.

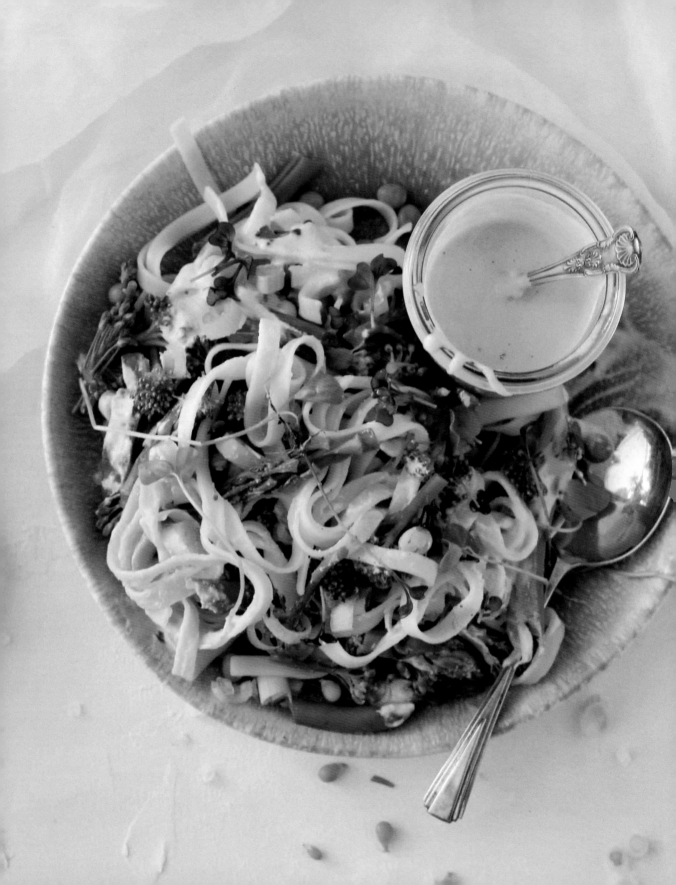

GREEN LEMONY VEGETABLE PASTA

PREPARATION: 20 MINUTES | SERVES 4–6

This is a lovely-looking pasta, and the fresh flavour of the vegetables and lemon shines through beautifully. Because the vegetables haven't been cooked to mush, they retain their fresh crunch and are therefore still full of enzymes and phytochemicals. Enjoy this dish — it's simple to make, delicious and healthy! I sometimes add a sprinkle of lemon zest over the final dish, to increase the fresh citrus flavour. You can also replace the pasta with rice noodles and add a sprinkling of chopped fresh red capsicum (bell pepper) just before serving — this adds a pretty colour and extra crunch. If you want to, add a dollop of sun-dried tomato pesto (see the tip on page 16) for extra flavour and nutrients, or any of the herb oils (see page 84).

250 grams/9 ounces (dried) gluten-free pasta

1 cup fresh peas

1–2 leeks or 1 onion, peeled and finely sliced

2 cups asparagus tips

1 medium broccoli, chopped into bite-sized pieces

2 cups green beans, halved

1½ cups savoury cashew nut cream (see options on page 32)

salt and pepper, to taste

1 bunch spring onions (shallots, scallions), finely chopped

¼ cup fresh lemon thyme, finely chopped, to garnish

Cook the pasta as per the package instructions.

Meanwhile, over boiling water, lightly steam the peas, leek or onion, asparagus, broccoli and beans for about 4 minutes.

When the pasta and vegetables are ready, carefully toss them together in a large bowl or serving dish. Add the savoury cashew cream and seasoning. Finely sprinkle the spring onion and thyme over the top to serve.

'MAC AND CHEESE' PASTA

PREPARATION: 25 MINUTES | SERVES 4–6

Although this dish contains no cheese, it is bright yellow and creamy, so is reminiscent of conventional mac and cheese. Using gluten-free pasta doesn't change the texture or taste, because this form of pasta tastes exactly like wheat-based pasta. You can use any shape of pasta, although I prefer the squiggly shapes because they hold onto the sauce well. Cook the sauce first, before you start cooking the pasta, because it will take longer than most pasta varieties to cook.

2 medium carrots, peeled and roughly chopped

1 cup peeled and cubed butternut pumpkin (squash), seeds removed

1 large onion, peeled and quartered

4–5 garlic cloves, peeled and roughly chopped

1 cup water

1 cup macadamia or cashew nuts

1½ cups rice milk

juice and rind of 1 large lemon

salt, to taste

250 grams/9 ounces (dried) gluten-free pasta

pesto of choice (see page 73)

In a saucepan, combine the carrot, pumpkin, onion and garlic. Pour over the water and place over a medium heat and cook for 20 minutes, or until the vegetables are tender, then remove from the heat.

Meanwhile, combine the nuts, rice milk and lemon juice in a blender (reserve the rind for later use). Blend until smooth and creamy.

Add the cooked vegetables to the blender and blend again until the mixture is creamy and smooth. Season with salt.

Cook the pasta as per the package instructions.

Pour the sauce over the pasta and serve immediately topped with the lemon rind and pesto of choice (see page 73).

Variations

Add a 500-gram (17-ounce) bottle of pasta sauce to the blended sauce before tossing with the pasta to increase nutrient density. Serve with pesto.

To make a delicious soup, simply increase the rice milk to 3 cups and add ½ cup tomato paste to the sauce, heating slowly. Serve with pesto.

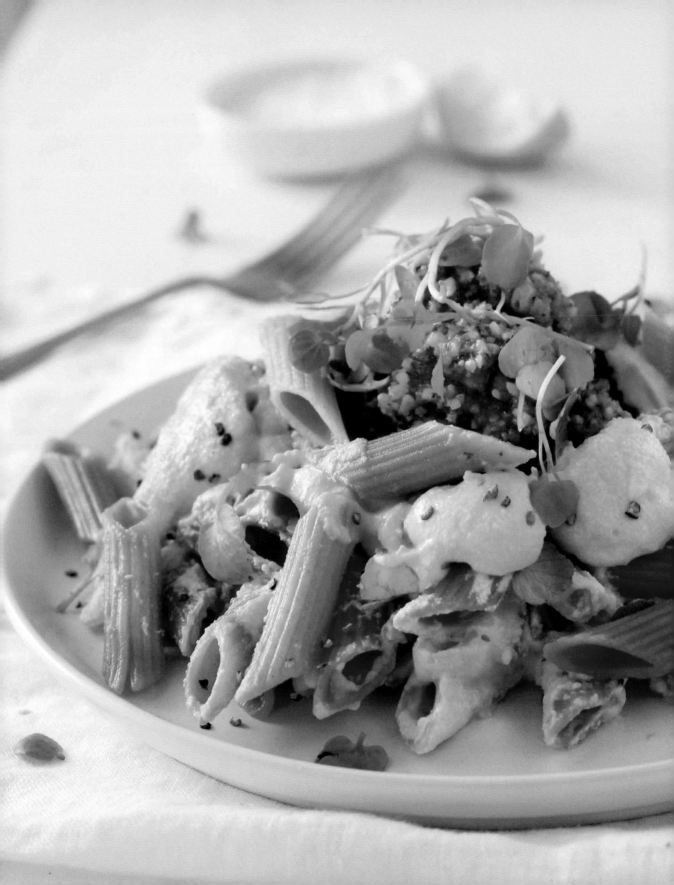

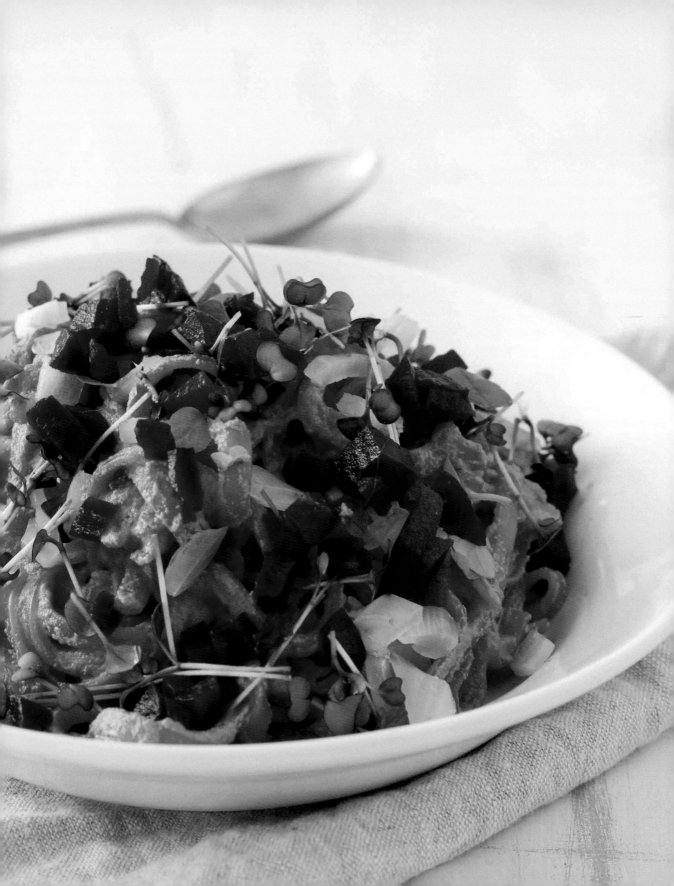

BEETROOT (BEET) PASTA

PREPARATION: 45 MINUTES | SERVES 6–8

This recipe takes a while to prepare, but when all the separate parts are done it's just tossed together and served immediately. The gorgeous colour and creamy sauce make it quite an impressive meal to look at — and to eat. The green herb oils (see page 84) look wonderful served on this dish, as do fresh sprouts.

Pasta

3 large beetroot (beets), scrubbed well, stems removed, and cubed

3 medium onions, peeled and quartered

1 head garlic, the small section on top sliced off to expose the cloves

250 grams/9 ounces (dried) gluten-free pasta

2 tablespoons olive oil

handful fresh basil or coriander (cilantro), roughly chopped, to garnish

Cream

1 cup macadamia nuts, soaked in water for an hour then drained and rinsed well

juice of 1 large lemon

1 cup water

2–3 tablespoons capers, rinsed well

salt and pepper, to taste (this will depend on whether the capers are salted)

Preheat the oven to 170°C/340°F. Line a baking tray (30 x 20 centimetres/12 x 8 inches) with baking paper.

On the baking tray, evenly spread the garlic head, beetroot and onions. Lay another sheet of baking paper over the vegetables and cover that layer with aluminum foil to allow the vegetables to steam-bake. Bake for 30 minutes.

Remove the tray from the oven and reduce the heat to 100°C/215°F. Remove the top layer of foil and baking paper, and return the vegetables to the oven for another 15 minutes.

Prepare the pasta according to the packet instructions so that it is cooked at the same time as the vegetables are ready to be removed from the oven.

To make the cream, in a blender combine the nuts, lemon juice and water. Blend on a high speed until thick and creamy. Add the capers and pulse briefly to roughly chop them.

Drain the pasta and return it to the pot. Toss with the olive oil, and then add the vegetables and cream, stirring well to combine. Sprinkle the basil or coriander over it, and serve immediately.

Variations

Add a dollop of pesto to increase nutrient density.

Replace the macadamia nuts with cashew nuts.

MEXICAN RE-FRIED BEANS

PREPARATION: 40 MINUTES | SERVES 4–6 WITH ACCOMPANIMENTS

Re-fried beans are a traditional Mexican dish made very simply using beans, onions, garlic and the spices cumin and coriander, freshly ground. Usually these ingredients are fried, but I only heat the spices in coconut oil and add the rest of the ingredients to simmer until they form a soft 'stew', which I mash with a potato masher until most of the beans are broken into smallish pieces. I then add freshly chopped coriander (cilantro) to this mixture just before serving. It doesn't look very exciting but the flavour and texture are great when served with fresh avocado salsa (see recipe on page 81), sour cream (see recipe on page 32) and fresh corn tortillas (see resources page 228).

3 tablespoons coconut oil or coconut cream

1 heaped teaspoon freshly ground cumin

1 heaped tablespoon freshly ground coriander

3 large white or red onions, peeled and sliced

6–7 large garlic cloves, peeled and finely sliced

5⅓ cups cooked beans (a combination of cannellini, borlotti and pinto beans works well) or 4 cans (425 grams/15 ounces each), drained

1 cup water, plus extra

salt, to taste

½ cup fresh coriander (cilantro), finely chopped, plus extra, to serve

6–8 fresh corn tortillas

avocado salsa (see recipe on page 81)

In a large saucepan, heat the coconut oil or cream slightly over a medium heat, then add the cumin and coriander and cook, stirring, for 2 minutes, until you can smell the spices. Add the onions, garlic and beans, and stir to coat with the spices. Lower the heat to a simmer and add the water, stirring well.

Add a little more water when the mixture sticks to the bottom of the saucepan, stirring well each time you add water. This process should take about 30 minutes, by which time the mixture will have become quite mushy and will be easy to scoop into a fresh tortilla.

Remove from the heat. Season with salt and stir the fresh coriander (cilantro) into the mixture. Place a few spoonfuls into a fresh tortilla and top it with fresh avocado salsa and some extra freshly chopped coriander.

Variation
Replace the tortillas with sturdy lettuce leaves and use them to wrap and hold the beans and sauces.

Beans

Beans are packed with protein along with most of the B vitamins, folate, iron potassium, phosphorous, magnesium and manganese. They contain lignins, also known as phyto-estrogens, which protect against different forms of cancer, as well as balancing hormone levels in the body. They are high in both insoluble and soluble fibre, which is great for gut and brain health. As a source of protein, they are also much less likely to contain high levels of environmental toxins, which conventionally grown animal products contain in large quantities; and because beans contain no fat, they can't store toxins in cell membranes like toxins are stored in animal forms of protein.

Lentils

Lentils are nutritious and versatile, as well as being quick to cook. They are one of our oldest foods, and signs of their use have been discovered as far back as 6750 BC in Iraq. Lentils contain protein, fibre and some B vitamins, as well as selenium, iron, zinc, manganese, phosphorous and folate. Combining them with rice or other grains in a meal creates a full complement of all the essential amino acids (protein) we require to stay healthy and build neurotransmitters (see page 6).

Rice

Rice has been one of humankind's most important foods throughout history. It is the staple food for two-thirds of the world's population today. Archaeological evidence suggests that rice has been feeding people for more than 5000 years. Brown rice is healthier than white rice because its outer layers of fibre have not been removed. Rice contains vitamins A, C, E and K as well as a number of B vitamins, folate, iron, magnesium, manganese and zinc. Brown rice also contains a variety of amino acids, the building blocks of protein, and brown rice soaked in water for a day contains three times as much lysine as white rice. Lysine is an essential amino acid needed for proper growth and development in children, and helps calcium absorption, tissue repair and collagen formation. Combining rice with a legume, such as lentils, creates a full complement of all the essential amino acids (protein) we require to stay healthy and build neurotransmitters (see page 6).

MUSHROOM AND LEMON 'RISOTTO'

PREPARATION: 45 MINUTES | SERVES 4–6

Although this isn't a real risotto, because I prefer to use brown rice rather than refined rice, it still has a lovely rice-and-cream flavour, so I've taken the liberty of calling it a risotto. The only downside to this meal is that you have to time it well so that you eat it as it has finished cooking — if you leave it to sit it will become mushy. As the cooking time will depend on the variety of brown rice you use, you will have to check when it's done after about 20 minutes, and may need to cook it for a little longer than suggested below.

Risotto

400-gram punnet (approximately 4 cups) button mushrooms (or a combination of various varieties), washed in a large bowl of water, rinsed and sliced

1 cup brown rice, soaked for 1 hour in enough water to cover the rice

1½ cups water blended with 3 peeled garlic cloves

1 large leek, washed and finely sliced, including the green stem

⅓ cup preserved lemon, rinsed well and finely sliced

small bunch parsley, finely sliced

¼ cup pine nuts

salt and pepper, to taste

fresh sprouts, to serve

Macadamia cream

juice of 1 large lemon

1 cup macadamia nuts

1 cup water

salt, to taste

Add the mushrooms to a medium saucepan and place over a high heat. Place a lid on the saucepan and cook for 2–3 minutes, then stir well. Reduce the heat and continue to cook, with the lid on, allowing the mushrooms to soften, sweat and release their moisture, which will take another 2–3 minutes.

Add the rice and stir to combine, then add the garlic water and allow to simmer for 40–45 minutes, stirring occasionally.

Meanwhile, to make the macadamia cream, combine all the ingredients in a blender and blend on high until smooth and creamy. Set aside as you finish making the risotto.

Add the leeks and cook for a further 2–3 minutes, then remove from the heat. Stir in the preserved lemon and parsley, and the macadamia cream and top with the pine nuts. Serve immediately.

(Depending on how salty the preserved lemon is, you may not have to add any salt to this dish.)

Variations

Replace the leek with 1 finely sliced medium onion.

Replace the preserved lemon with 1 tablespoon finely sliced lemon rind.

JASMINE RICE, MUSHROOM AND LENTIL PILAF/SALAD

PREPARATION: 45 MINUTES | SERVES 4–6 AS A SIDE DISH

This is an adaptable meal — you can serve it as a warm salad or as a main meal, depending on what you feel like and how many people you are serving. Either way, it is very simple to prepare, and makes great leftovers for lunch the next day. I like to serve it on a bed of extra green leaves, such as watercress, to increase nutrient content.

1 cup jasmine rice

1 tablespoon dried Italian herbs

1 teaspoon dried garlic

1 large punnet (about 400 grams or 4 cups) mushrooms

1⅓ cups cooked lentils, or 1 can (425 grams/15 ounces) lentils, drained

4–5 spring onions (shallots, scallions), finely sliced

3–4 cups baby kale or baby spinach leaves, finely chopped

1 bottle (250 grams/8 ounces) artichoke hearts, drained and finely sliced

½ cup sun-dried tomatoes, finely sliced

¼ cup fresh parsley or basil, finely sliced and a few sprigs left to garnish

Rinse the rice well under running water. Place rice, herbs and garlic in a saucepan with 2 cups of water, bring to the boil and simmer for 15 minutes, then remove from the heat and set aside for 10 minutes, keeping the lid on.

Meanwhile, place the mushrooms in a large saucepan over medium heat. Sauté in their juices, stirring occasionally, for 10–15 minutes, until they are cooked and have absorbed most of their juices.

Stir the lentils into the warm mushroom mixture. Add the cooked rice, spring onions, kale or spinach leaves, artichoke hearts and sun-dried tomatoes, tossing to combine them well.

Stir in the finely sliced herbs and leave to sit for 5 minutes for the flavours to develop fully, then serve topped with a few extra basil or parsley sprigs.

Variations

Toss in some spicy baked sweet potato cubes (see page 134) to turn this into a main meal.

Replace the jasmine rice with brown basmati rice and cook for 45 minutes, then remove from heat, keeping the lid on, and stand for 10 minutes before fluffing.

Tip

If you want rice to remain separate and not stick together, add a large squeeze of lemon juice to the rice and water before cooking.

LENTIL AND RICE PANCAKES/WRAPS

PREPARATION: 45 MINUTES (PLUS OVERNIGHT SOAKING) | SERVES 6–8
(OR 10–12 IF YOU MAKE SMALLER PANCAKES)

These are amazingly simple to make if you soak the rice and lentils the night before. And if you soak the full amount, you can freeze half, depending on how many you want to serve, so the next time you make these pancakes you only have to defrost the rice and and lentils, not soak them. They are very versatile, because you can add whatever fillings you have on hand (see variations below).

1½ cups brown rice

1½ cups whole red lentils

water, to soak

5 cups water, extra

2 garlic cloves

1 teaspoon herb salt

½ cup finely chopped coriander (cilantro) or parsley

½ cup peeled and grated carrots

1 tablespoon coconut oil

Soak the brown rice and red lentils overnight. Use enough water to keep them covered.

Preheat the oven to 50°C/120°F or its 'warm' setting.

Drain the rice and lentils well until the water runs clear, then combine with the water, garlic and herb salt in a blender and blend on high until the mixture is smooth and creamy. (If you are using half the mixture, halve the other ingredients.)

Transfer the mixture to a large bowl and add the coriander or parsley and the carrots.

Heat the coconut oil in a medium non-stick frying pan. Using a ½-cup measure (which makes 20 pancakes), add the mixture to the pan and tilt the pan to spread the mixture around the pan. (Use a smaller measure to make smaller pancakes.)

Let the pancake cook for about 3 minutes while bubbles form on the surface, then turn it over and cook for about 2 minutes. Remove it from the pan and place it on a large plate in the oven to keep warm while you repeat the process with the remaining mixture.

Variations
Serve filled with the spicy chickpea (garbanzo bean) and tomato stew (see recipe on page 168), or with the baked tofu (see recipe on page 116) and a large green salad, as well as a combination of any of the following: spicy baked sweet potato cubes (page 134), spiced cauliflower (see recipe on page 177), avocado salsa (see recipe on page 81), salsa verde (see recipe on page 82) or turmeric macadamia mayonnaise (see recipe on page 72) and lemon/lime wedges.

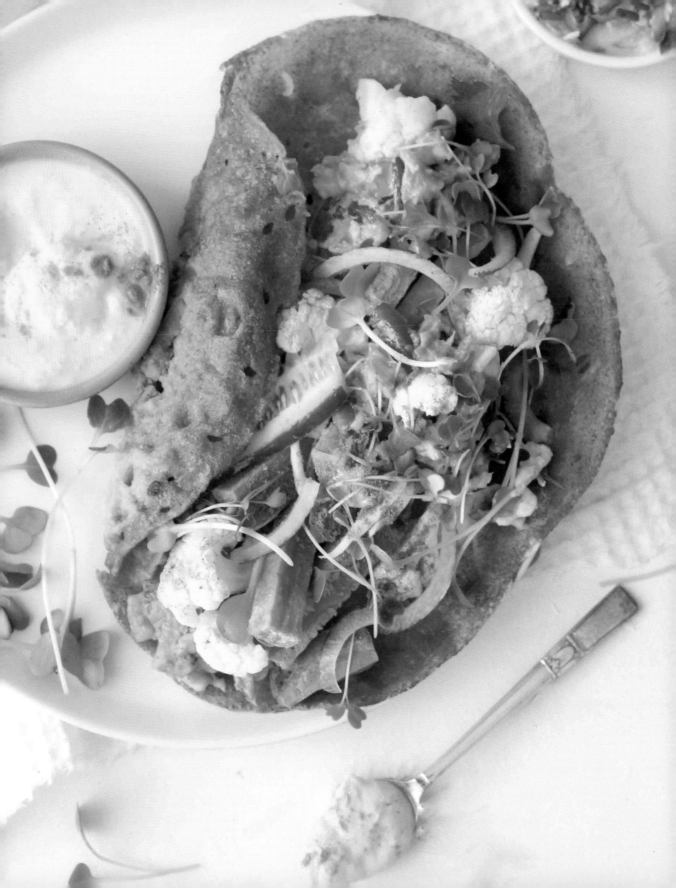

SPICY CHICKPEA (GARBANZO BEAN) AND TOMATO STEW

PREPARATION: 30 MINUTES | SERVES 4–5

This is a very simple stew to throw together, which you can serve with the gluten-free flat bread (see recipe on page 120), rice, millet or quinoa. It also makes a great filling for the lentil and rice pancakes (see recipe on page 166), and it easily converts into a chunky, thick soup that you can serve with a dollop of green pesto (see recipe on page 73).

2 tablespoons coconut oil

2 tablespoons brown or yellow mustard seeds

2 medium onions, peeled and roughly chopped

2 garlic cloves, finely chopped

1½ tablespoons mild curry powder (see page 85)

2⅔ cups cooked chickpeas (garbanzo bean), or 2 cans (425 grams/15 ounces each)

½ cup tomato paste

¾ cup water

salt and pepper, to taste

½ small bunch basil, finely chopped, to serve

Heat the coconut oil in a large saucepan over medium heat and add the mustard seeds. Put the lid on, and when you hear the sound of popping, immediately remove the saucepan from the heat, shake to distribute the heat and wait until the popping subsides, which will take 2–3 minutes.

Return the saucepan to the heat, and add the onions, garlic and curry powder. Stir well until you can smell the lovely curry spices that the heat has released, and then add the chickpeas, tomato paste and water. Put the lid back on the saucepan, and allow the stew to simmer for about 30 minutes, until all the ingredients are well cooked.

Sprinkle the basil over the top to serve.

Variation
To convert this stew into a tasty soup, add 1 cup of water and 1 can of coconut milk (400 millilitres/13 fluid ounces).

MILLET AND KALE STIR-FRY

PREPARATION: 20 MINUTES | SERVES 4

Although the title for this recipe doesn't sound very tasty, the dish is! It's also really simple to throw together, and with the peanut satay sauce (see recipe on page 78) it's really tasty, nutrient dense and full of fibre. When I cook millet I always make double the quantity, because it's even simpler to throw this dish together when you have a packet of frozen millet at hand — just remember to defrost it before you need to use it.

5 tablespoons coconut oil

2 large onions, peeled and sliced

5 large garlic cloves, peeled and finely sliced

4 tablespoons finely ground fresh ginger (see page 15 for the simplest way to use fresh ginger) or 2 teaspoons ground ginger

2 cups cooked millet (see page 28 for cooking instructions)

1 punnet (about 4 cups) baby kale

salt, to taste

1 cup peanut satay sauce (see recipe on page 78)

½ cup roughly chopped peanuts, to serve

Heat the coconut oil in a large wok over medium heat. Add the onions, garlic and ginger, and stir to combine well. Simmer until the onions are soft, and then add the millet and kale and stir to combine and wilt the leaves. Cook for about 3 minutes to lightly cook the leaves and then season with salt.

Serve with the peanut satay sauce and top each serve with peanuts.

Variations

Stir through ½ cup finely chopped coriander (cilantro) and top with a dollop of green pesto (see recipe on page 73).

Stir through the baked tofu (see recipe on page 116) to increase nutrient density.

Millet

Millet is a small yellow grain that has been cultivated in Africa and Asia for the past 10,000 years, being one of the most important food staples in these areas. It is an easy replacement for couscous, because the grains can also be fluffed up and it even looks similar, due to the shape of the small pellet-like grains. It contains complex carbohydrates, fibre and protein, as well as magnesium and a good quantity of iron, and zinc, and is rich in B vitamins, all important brain nutrients.

CARAMELIZED ONION, CAPSICUM (BELL PEPPER) AND CHICKPEA (GARBANZO BEAN) STEW

PREPARATION: 10 MINUTES (PLUS 45 MINUTES COOKING TIME) | SERVES 4–6

Although you can serve this tasty dish on rice, quinoa or millet, I like to serve it with a wedge of sun-dried tomato and sweet-corn polenta (see recipe on page 173). It's really simple to assemble, but you need to be patient and let it cook for the allotted time so that you end up with caramelized onions and the capsicums (bell peppers) get a chance to soften nicely.

1⅓ cups cooked chickpeas (garbanzo beans), or 1 can (425 grams/15 ounces), drained

2 garlic cloves, peeled and finely sliced

2 medium onions, peeled and thickly sliced

2 large red capsicums (bell peppers), halved, seeded and chopped

2 teaspoons smoked paprika

¼ cup water

2 tablespoons olive oil

1 tablespoon lemon juice

1 tablespoon maple or rice syrup

salt and pepper, to taste

¼ cup salted capers, washed and drained well

¼ cup fresh basil, finely chopped

In a large saucepan, combine the chickpeas, garlic, onion, capsicum, paprika, water, olive oil, lemon juice and syrup, and season with salt and pepper. Place over a high heat and bring to the boil, then reduce the heat to a simmer and cook for 20–25 minutes, until the onions are caramelized and the capsicums are soft and juicy.

Top with the capers and basil and serve on your grain of choice, or on slices of polenta.

Variation
Replace the capers with a dollop of green pesto (see recipe on page 73).

Tip
Lightly crush the chickpeas with a fork before adding them to the sauce, because they will absorb more of the sauce's flavour.

Paprika is made from dried and ground sweet red capsicums (bell peppers) or chilli peppers. Traditional Hungarian and South American cooking calls for the use of paprika, although it is now used around the world. It ranges from mild to hot, depending on the type of fresh produce used. Paprika is antibacterial, as well as very high in the antioxidants vitamin C and A, along with vitamin E. It also contains the 'eye' nutrients lutein and zeaxanthin. Research indicates that foods from the capsicum family may improve circulation, normalize blood pressure and aid digestion. However, commercially dried peppers are exposed to very high temperatures, so choose organic, naturally dried paprika. It deteriorates quickly, getting darker the longer it is kept, so buy it in small quantities.

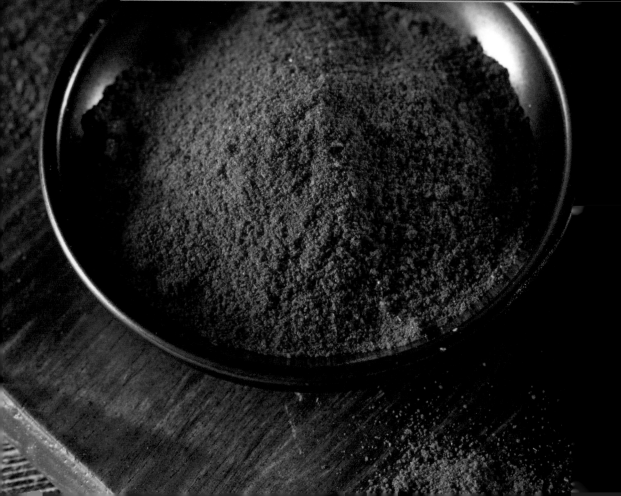

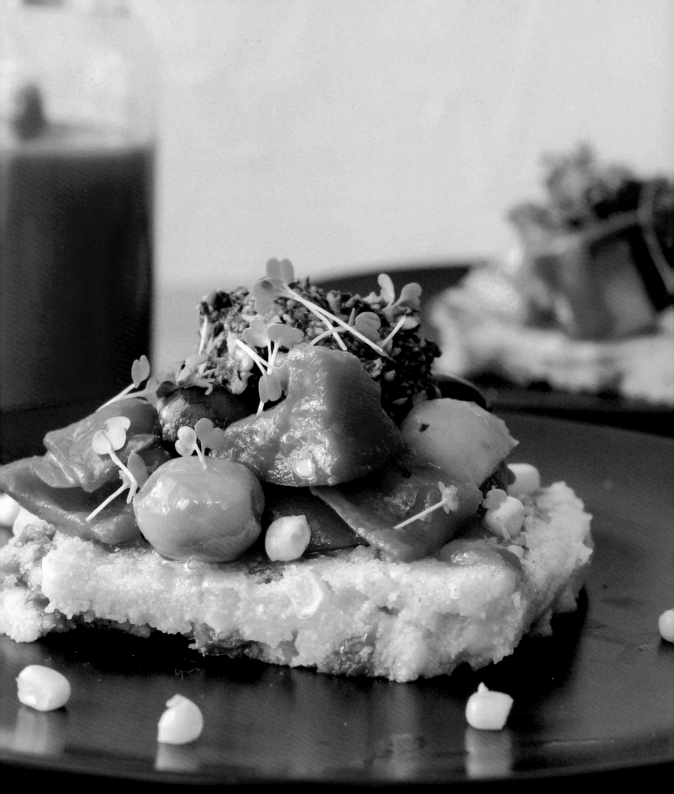

SUN-DRIED TOMATO AND SWEET-CORN POLENTA WITH VEGETABLES
(RECIPE CONTINUES OVERLEAF)

PREPARATION: 45 MINUTES | SERVES 6

Sailing along the Turkish coast, we had the delightful experience of coming into a port and being met by a little boat offering fresh vegetables for sale. They had lovely fresh tomatoes, capsicums (bell peppers), marrows (zucchini/courgette) and enormous eggplants (aubergine) — all wonderful summer vegetables. We decided to use them for lunch, but we only had polenta, some frozen sweet corn and sun-dried tomatoes left in our pantry. This is what we came up with. The fresh flavours of the Mediterranean summer shine through! When we got home I added some spring onions (shallots, scallions), asparagus and fresh basil to this basic recipe. You can sprinkle it with basil oil (see recipe on page 84) or a dollop of sun-dried tomato pesto (see the tip on page 73) to serve. Enjoy!

1 quantity basic tomato sauce (see recipe on page 62), or use a good quality, bottled, organic pasta sauce

1 cup polenta

2½ cups water

1 cup sweet corn or 2 fresh sweet corn, kernels sliced off

5 spring onions (shallots, scallions), finely chopped

1 cup sun-dried tomatoes (if in oil, drain and retain oil), finely chopped

½ cup finely chopped fresh basil

salt, to taste

1 medium eggplant (aubergine), washed, tops removed and sliced into strips (degorge if necessary — see page 152)

1 red capsicum (bell pepper) and 1 yellow capsicum, seeded and sliced into 6 strips each

3 tablespoons water

3 tablespoons olive oil

6 asparagus spears, trimmed (optional)

fresh basil, to garnish (optional)

2–3 tablespoons olive oil, extra

½ cup black or green olives, to serve

1 cup green pesto (see recipe on page 73), to serve

2–3 tablespoons olive oil, extra to serve

SUN-DRIED TOMATO AND SWEET-CORN POLENTA WITH VEGETABLES
(CONTINUED)

Preheat the oven to 160°C/320°F. Coat an oven-proof dish (20 x 25 centimetres/8 x 10 inches) with olive oil.

Prepare the tomato sauce.

To make the polenta, pour the water into a large saucepan, cover with a lid and place over a high heat. Bring to the boil, then reduce the heat and add the polenta, stirring well to ensure no lumps form. Add the sweet corn, onions, sun-dried tomatoes, basil and salt and cook the polenta for 30 minutes, stirring frequently.

Pour the cooked polenta into the oiled oven-proof dish. (If you use instant polenta, follow the instructions on the packet and then continue.)

Cook the eggplant and capsicum in water for about 30 minutes until soft and juicy, then add the olive oil, stirring to coat.

Place the asparagus in a bowl, and pour boiling water over the top. Leave the asparagus in the water for 1 minute, then drain.

Slice the polenta into six pieces and place each piece on a separate plate, on a couple of tablespoons of tomato sauce. Serve each topped with 1 tablespoon of the tomato sauce, equal amounts of the vegetable mixture, asparagus, olives and pesto, and drizzle with extra olive oil, topping with the basil.

Variation
Drizzle with basil oil (see recipe on page 84) and a few basil sprigs.

SPICY SWEET POTATO 'CHIPS'

PREPARATION: 30 MINUTES | MAKES 2–3 CUPS

Most of the sweet potato 'chips' served in restaurants have either been fried in very hot oil or covered in oil and baked in a hot oven, both variations not the best for keeping our brains healthy. In this version, we bake the sweet potatoes without anything added, and then cover them with a great olive-oil based sauce after they are removed from the oven, yielding a very tasty and much healthier version, because olive oil gets damaged when heated in the oven. I generally add about ¼ cup of freshly chopped coriander (cilantro) too — it adds nutrients, flavour and colour. Serve with fresh avocado salsa (see recipe on page 81) or red capsicum (bell pepper) hummus (see recipe on page 75) and with the pecan and bean burgers (page 147).

4 sweet potatoes, washed well, tops and bottoms cut off, chopped into the shape of fries or simply cubed

½ cup olive oil

1 tablespoon ground cumin

1 tablespoon ground coriander

1 tablespoon ground paprika

juice of 1 lemon

2 garlic cloves, peeled and crushed

fresh coriander (cilantro), chopped

Preheat the oven to 160°C/320°F. Line a baking tray with baking paper.

Spread the sweet potato evenly over the baking tray. Bake for 30 minutes.

To make the sauce, combine the olive oil, cumin, ground coriander, paprika, lemon, garlic and fresh coriander in a bowl. Mix well, and then pour over the chips as you remove them from the oven.

EXTRA TIPS

When preparing a meal that requires a grain, such as millet, quinoa or rice (see page 29 for cooking millet and quinoa) I like to enhance the nutrient density, texture, colour and flavour of the meal by doing any of the following:

- Add 1 cup chopped fresh herbs, such as basil, coriander (cilantro), dill or parsley to cooked grains.

- Chop up some preserved lemon, with the pulp removed, and add ⅓ cup lightly crushed almonds.

- Grate some frozen ginger (see page 15) and chop up some shelled pistachio nuts and toss through the grain before serving.

- Make a 'jewelled' grain dish by adding some grated carrots, steamed corn pieces, steamed peas, finely sliced spring onions (shallots scallions) including their green leaves, chopped red capsicum (bell peppers), finely sliced fresh herbs and pomegranate seeds.

- Remember to add any of the condiments, such as the lemon rind, herbs, sun-dried tomatoes, onion, beetroot (beets), spicy baked sweet potato chips or cubes (see pages 175) or grated ginger (see page 15) to any grains to enhance the flavour and nutrient density of meals served with them.

OTHER IDEAS

- For a tasty vegetable dish, toss some pesto with oven-roasted vegetables, such as baked cauliflower, after removing them from the oven.

- Cook gluten-free pasta according to directions and toss with pesto and baked sweet potato (see page 175).

- Cook gluten-free pasta according to directions and toss with tomato sauce (see recipes on pages 62 and 64), finely sliced capers, drained artichoke hearts, sun-dried tomato (see page 16), finely sliced basil and a dollop of pesto.

- Cook gluten-free pasta according to directions and toss with lightly steamed green beans, finely sliced preserved lemon, finely sliced dill, crushed garlic and savoury cashew nut cream (see options on page 32).

- Cook gluten-free pasta according to directions and toss with a variety of mushrooms cooked in their own juices (see page 165), finely sliced spring onions (shallots, scallions), crushed walnuts and pesto.

- Cook rice, turn heat to low and toss in baby peas and sliced baby spinach along with finely sliced spring onions and savoury cashew cream and serve with a dollop of sun-dried tomato pesto (see the tip on page 73).

- Replace any grain with 'magical' cauliflower grains: use a head of washed cauliflower, which you either grate or cut into chunks and process using the pulse option, in batches, until it is broken down into grain-sized granules. Remove largish chunks of the stalk, then lightly steam or cook for about 5 minutes. Serve immediately.

- Top spicy cooked quinoa with roasted vegetables (sweet potatoes, sliced fennel bulbs, quartered onions, baby tomatoes) and top with drained chickpeas (garbanzo beans) and almonds or pistachio, and any of the tomato sauces (see pages 62 and 64), or the paprika-spice sauce on page 65.

- Combine 1 cup cooked millet (see page 29) with 1 cup (or can) cooked, drained lentils and toss with ½ cup pesto (see page 73) and 2 cups baked sweet potato (see page 175). Top with a dollop of avocado salsa (see page 81) or salsa verde (see page 82) for a very simple, quick meal.

- Make a 'meal in a bowl' by combining a few cooked items such as cooked quinoa (see page 29), lentil dahl (see page 124), avocado salsa (see recipe on page 81) and cucumber cooler (see recipe on page 143) with a handful of sprouts and rocket (arugula) leaves and a lovely salad dressing. This is a super-simple way to make a satisfying meal in a few minutes.

- Make spiced cauliflower florets by breaking the cauliflower into small florets and tossing with coconut oil, curry powder and salt and bake at 160°C/320°F on a baking tray lined with baking paper for about 15 minutes. Use with the lentil and rice pancakes (page 166) or tossed into a salad for extra nutrients.

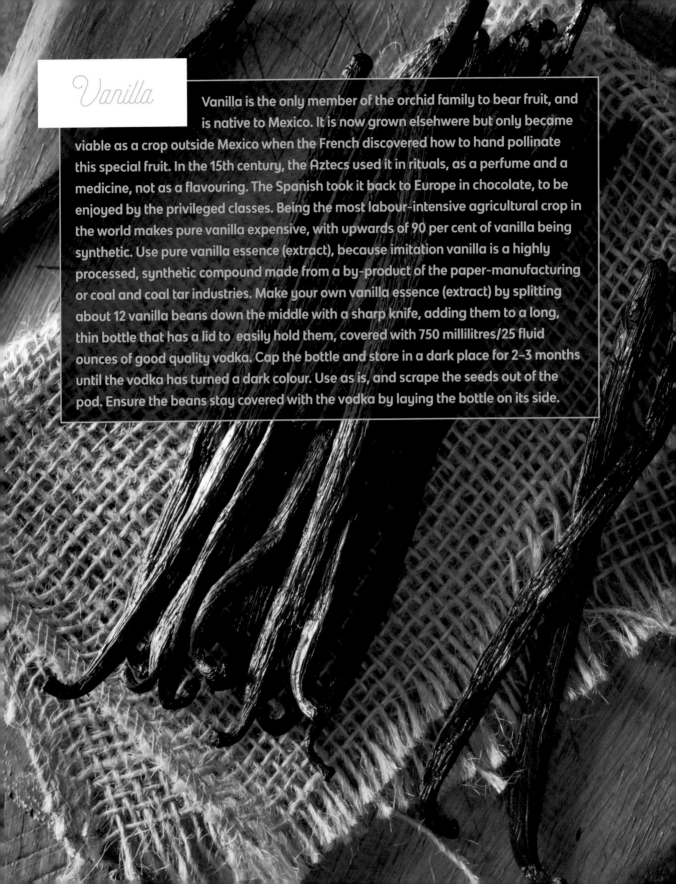

Vanilla

Vanilla is the only member of the orchid family to bear fruit, and is native to Mexico. It is now grown elsehwere but only became viable as a crop outside Mexico when the French discovered how to hand pollinate this special fruit. In the 15th century, the Aztecs used it in rituals, as a perfume and a medicine, not as a flavouring. The Spanish took it back to Europe in chocolate, to be enjoyed by the privileged classes. Being the most labour-intensive agricultural crop in the world makes pure vanilla expensive, with upwards of 90 per cent of vanilla being synthetic. Use pure vanilla essence (extract), because imitation vanilla is a highly processed, synthetic compound made from a by-product of the paper-manufacturing or coal and coal tar industries. Make your own vanilla essence (extract) by splitting about 12 vanilla beans down the middle with a sharp knife, adding them to a long, thin bottle that has a lid to easily hold them, covered with 750 millilitres/25 fluid ounces of good quality vodka. Cap the bottle and store in a dark place for 2–3 months until the vodka has turned a dark colour. Use as is, and scrape the seeds out of the pod. Ensure the beans stay covered with the vodka by laying the bottle on its side.

DESSERTS AND TREATS

When you make the decision to eat according to your health it's easy to end up feeling deprived, especially with regards to sweet treats. And the brain doesn't like that feeling at all. However, if you have the basic ingredients for healthy snacks in your pantry, then it's really easy to make sweet treats in as little as 10 minutes and baked treats in less than half an hour. Keep in mind, though, that these foods are treats and should not be consumed in vast quantities — although, being nutrient dense and containing good fats they are very satisfying and it's therefore hard to over-indulge! Remember, it's best to avoid treats containing chocolate after 4 p.m., because the theobromine in chocolate is a stimulating compound and can interfere with sleep.

EMMA'S BANANA CHOCOLATE 'PIE'

PREPARATION: 10 MINUTES | MAKES ABOUT 10 SLICES

This is a simple yet delicious and rich dessert that can be made quickly. It gets rather thick when refrigerated, which makes it similar to a cheesecake in consistency, but needs no baking or complicated steps. It's my daughter's favourite treat. Enjoy!

2 ripe bananas, peeled and roughly chopped

½ cup tahini

4 tablespoons raw cacao powder

¼ cup coconut nectar, or maple or rice syrup

1½ teaspoons agar-agar powder

½ teaspoon pure vanilla essence (vanilla extract)

pinch of salt

Combine all the ingredients in a blender and blend until the mixture becomes hot, which activates the agar-agar powder.

Pour the mixture into a glass container (approximately 9 x 6 centimetres/3½ x 2¼ inches) and refrigerate for 4 hours.

When the mixture has set, slice it into equal slices with a warm knife, and keep leftovers in an airtight glass container in the refrigerator for up to a week.

Variation
Replace the tahini with peanut butter for another lovely flavour.

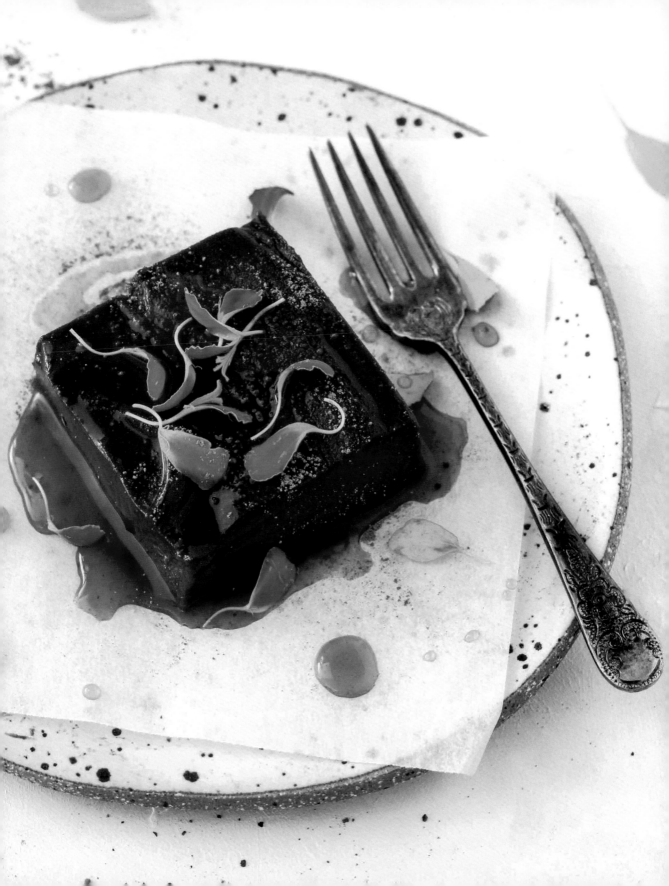

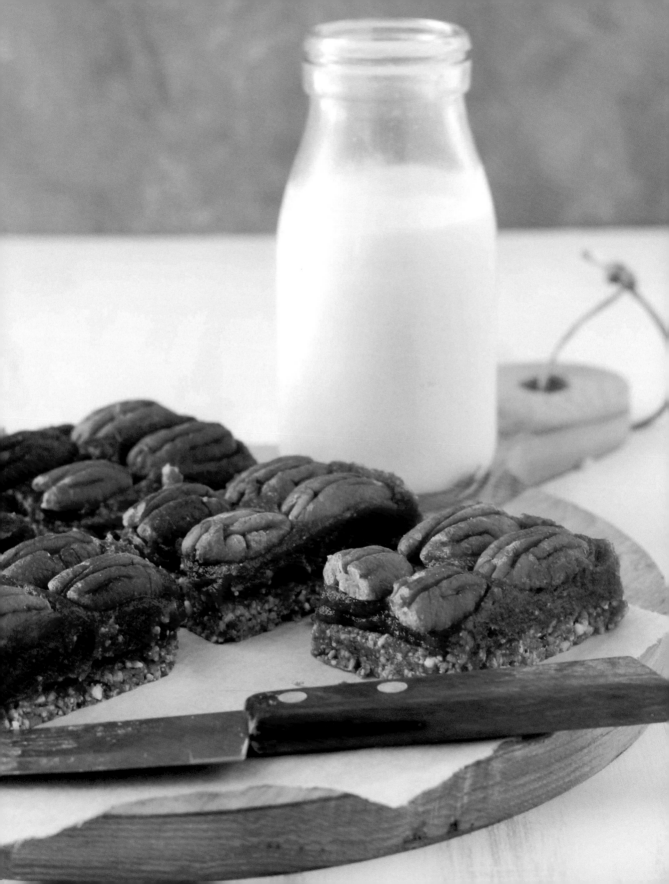

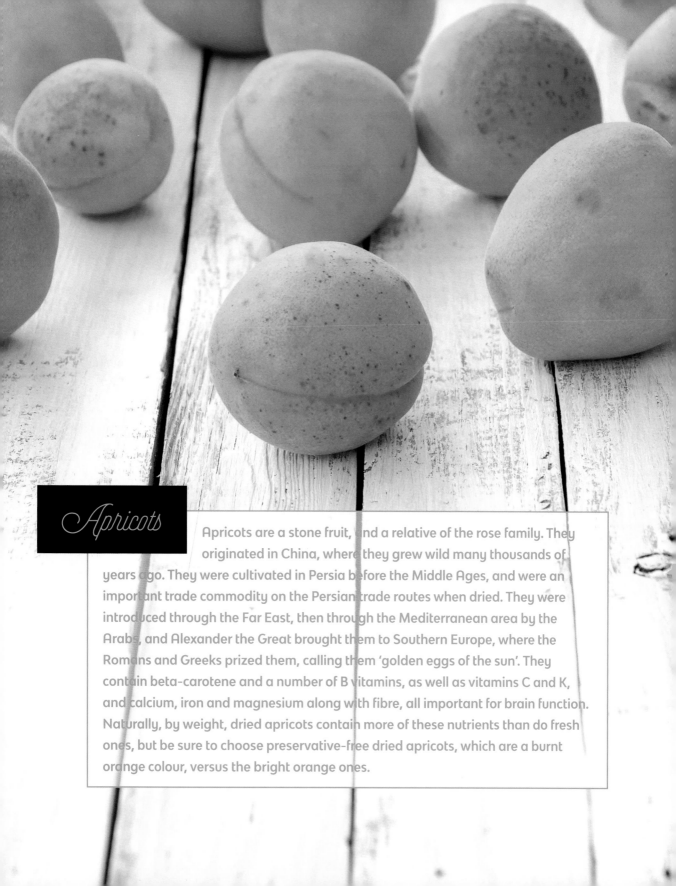

Apricots

Apricots are a stone fruit, and a relative of the rose family. They originated in China, where they grew wild many thousands of years ago. They were cultivated in Persia before the Middle Ages, and were an important trade commodity on the Persian trade routes when dried. They were introduced through the Far East, then through the Mediterranean area by the Arabs, and Alexander the Great brought them to Southern Europe, where the Romans and Greeks prized them, calling them 'golden eggs of the sun'. They contain beta-carotene and a number of B vitamins, as well as vitamins C and K, and calcium, iron and magnesium along with fibre, all important for brain function. Naturally, by weight, dried apricots contain more of these nutrients than do fresh ones, but be sure to choose preservative-free dried apricots, which are a burnt orange colour, versus the bright orange ones.

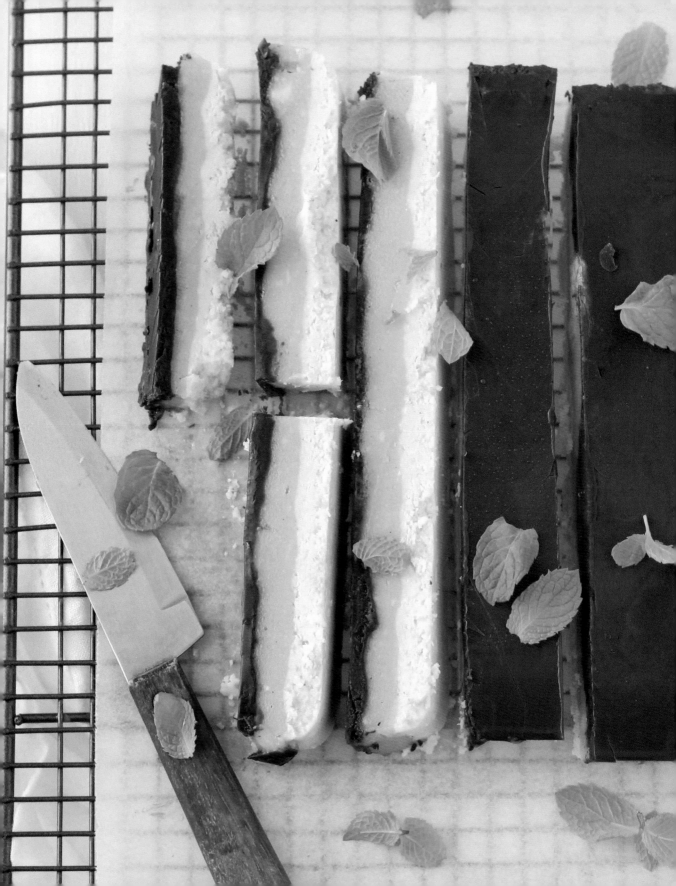

CHOCOLATE MINT SLICE

PREPARATION: 20 MINUTES | MAKES 24

This is simple to make, and very tasty, but there are a few steps to follow and it's quite messy to consume. If you freeze it before serving it's a lot easier to eat! I make each part separately, and then add it to the tray and put it in the freezer. In this way, each part is really cold when I add the next layer. This means it's ready to be eaten when you add the last layer, which just solidifies as you spread it.

Crust
1½ cups desiccated coconut

¾ cup cashews

1 tablespoon coconut oil

pinch of salt

Peppermint filling
1¼ cup macadamia nuts

2 tablespoons maple or rice syrup

3 tablespoons coconut oil

¼ teaspoon pure vanilla essence (vanilla extract)

6 drops organic peppermint essential oil

Chocolate topping
½ cup melted (50 grams/1¾ ounces) raw cacao butter

3 tablespoons raw cacao powder

3 tablespoons maple syrup or rice syrup

¼ teaspoon pure vanilla essence (vanilla extract)

To make the crust, combine the coconut, cashews, coconut oil and salt in a food processor and blend until they form soft crumbs. Press the mixture into a baking tray (20 x 6 centimetres/8 x 2¼ inches) and place the tray in the freezer while you prepare the filling.

To make the peppermint filling, combine the macadamia nuts, syrup, coconut oil, vanilla and peppermint oil in a blender or food processor. Blend until the mixture is mostly smooth but with a few remaining macadamia chunks.

Remove the crust from the freezer and spread the peppermint mixture over the cold crust. Return the tray to the freezer while you prepare the topping.

To make the chocolate topping, melt the cacao butter in a saucepan over a very low heat, slowly adding the cacao powder, syrup and vanilla. Stir well to remove any lumps, and then remove from the heat.

Remove the crust from the freezer and pour the topping over the frozen peppermint and crust layers, spreading evenly. Return to the freezer for 30 minutes, until the topping has set.

When the topping has set, use a hot knife to slice, and serve immediately.

Store leftovers in an airtight glass container in the refrigerator for up to 10 days.

CHOCOLATE CLUSTERS

PREPARATION: 15 MINUTES | MAKES 24

This is my go-to chunky chocolate treat — it's really simple to make and is nutrient dense, so one or two are super-satisfying. I love it with the variation of apricot slices, and dried cherries are wonderful too. The addition of psyllium husks means that it contains extra fibre, so you won't be able to eat too many!

10 small dates, pitted, or 4–5
   Medjool dates, pitted

½ cup Brazil nuts

½ cup cashew nuts

1 cup desiccated coconut

1 tablespoon psyllium husks

120 grams (4 ounces) dark
   chocolate (70 per cent)

Line a baking tray with baking paper.

Combine the dates, nuts, coconut and psyllium in a food processor and blend for 2–3 minutes, until well chopped and mixed, scraping the bowl down if necessary.

Melt the chocolate in a large bowl over a saucepan that contains water simmering over a low heat. Remove from the heat and stir the date and nut mixture into the melted chocolate.

Drop spoonfuls of the mixture evenly onto the baking tray, until you have used all the mixture. Refrigerate until the clusters are set, which will take about half an hour, then transfer them to a glass container with an airtight lid, and store in the refrigerator for up to 2 weeks.

Variations

Replace the dates with ½ cup finely sliced dried apricots or ½ cup dried blueberries, cherries or cranberries.

Replace the cashew nuts with macadamia nuts.

For a spicy version, add ¼ teaspoon cinnamon and ¼ teaspoon nutmeg.

Tip

Instead of all the bother of using a double boiler to melt chocolate, I have found that simply adding the quantity of chocolate required to an oven-safe glass container and inserting the container into an oven heated to 50°C/120°F (or on its 'warm' setting) and then turned off, for about 20 minutes, will melt the chocolate beautifully.

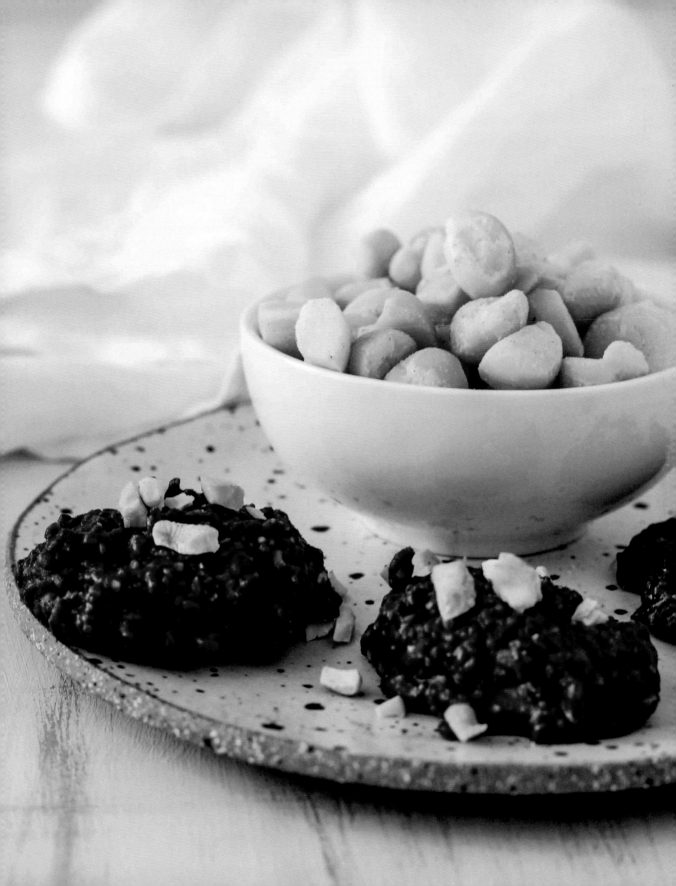

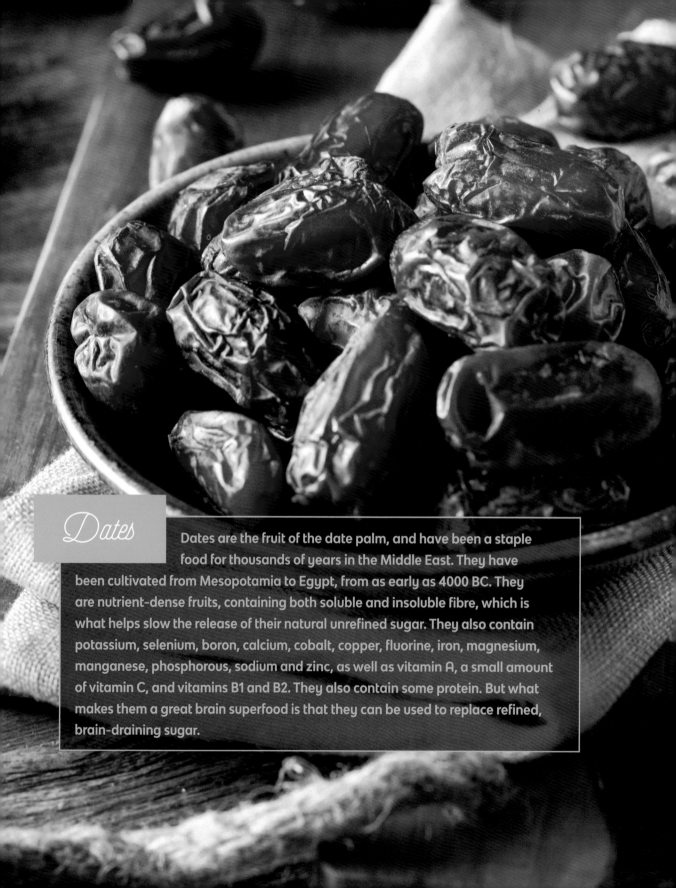

Dates

Dates are the fruit of the date palm, and have been a staple food for thousands of years in the Middle East. They have been cultivated from Mesopotamia to Egypt, from as early as 4000 BC. They are nutrient-dense fruits, containing both soluble and insoluble fibre, which is what helps slow the release of their natural unrefined sugar. They also contain potassium, selenium, boron, calcium, cobalt, copper, fluorine, iron, magnesium, manganese, phosphorous, sodium and zinc, as well as vitamin A, a small amount of vitamin C, and vitamins B1 and B2. They also contain some protein. But what makes them a great brain superfood is that they can be used to replace refined, brain-draining sugar.

ALMOND, TAHINI AND DATE PROTEIN SNACKS

PREPARATION: 10 MINUTES | MAKES 24

This is another quick and easy snack that you could whip up at a moment's notice.

1 cup almonds

1 cup desiccated coconut

8 large Medjool dates, pitted

¼ cup tahini

1–2 tablespoons coconut oil

2 tablespoons sesame seeds

Grind together the almonds, coconut, dates, tahini and coconut oil in a food processor until they resemble small breadcrumbs — use just enough coconut oil to allow the mixture to stick together into a ball.

If you prefer a slice, transfer the contents into a glass baking dish (9 x 5 centimetres/3½ x 2 inches) and press down firmly. Sprinkle the sesame seeds over the mixture and cut into even-sized squares or triangles, and refrigerate until set. Alternatively, using your hands, roll the mixture into balls, dip into the sesame seeds, and refrigerate until set, which will take a couple of hours.

Variation
Replace almonds with cashew nuts.

WHITE CHOCOLATE MOUSSE

PREPARATION: 10 MINUTES | SERVES 4–6

This is the simplest and most stunning dessert to make, because all it requires is the ingredients, a powerful blender, some patience and gorgeous fresh berries. Serve it with fresh blueberries, cherries or raspberries and a sprinkle of dark raw cacao powder. If you want to make an amazing dessert, halve this recipe and the dark chocolate mousse (see recipe on page 208) and make layers of these two stunning desserts in glasses, also topping with fresh berries.

½ cup melted (55 grams/ 2 ounces) raw cacao butter

1½ cups cashew nuts

2 tablespoons coconut nectar, or maple or rice syrup, plus a few extra teaspoons to serve

1 cup coconut milk

1 teaspoon pure vanilla essence (vanilla extract)

1 cup fresh berries, to serve

Melt the cacao butter over very low heat for 2–3 minutes then transfer to a blender. Add the cashew nuts, coconut nectar or syrup, coconut milk and vanilla, and blend until smooth and creamy.

Transfer the mixture to a flat, glass rectangular dish (24 x 19 centimetres/9½ x 7½ inches) or into individual glasses, and refrigerate for 5–6 hours.

When the mousse is ready, use an ice-cream scoop to serve, or serve in glasses, and top with fresh berries.

Raspberries

Raspberries have been eaten in Europe since prehistoric times, with cultivation dates going back to the 17th century in England. They thrive in cool, damp climates (even in Alaska) while in North America they are cultivated from an indigenous species, suited to the prevailing dry and hot conditions. They are a member of the rose family and contain vitamin B2 and B3, vitamin C as well as potassium and have potent antioxidant power in their bright red colour. They contain one of the highest amounts of fibre found in any whole food, with up to 20 per cent of their weight being made up of fibre.

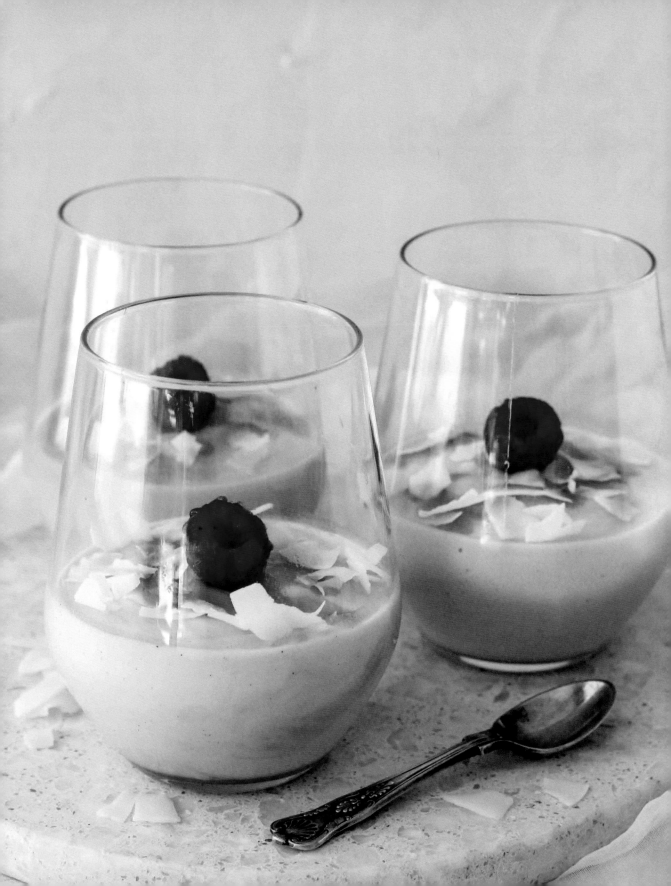

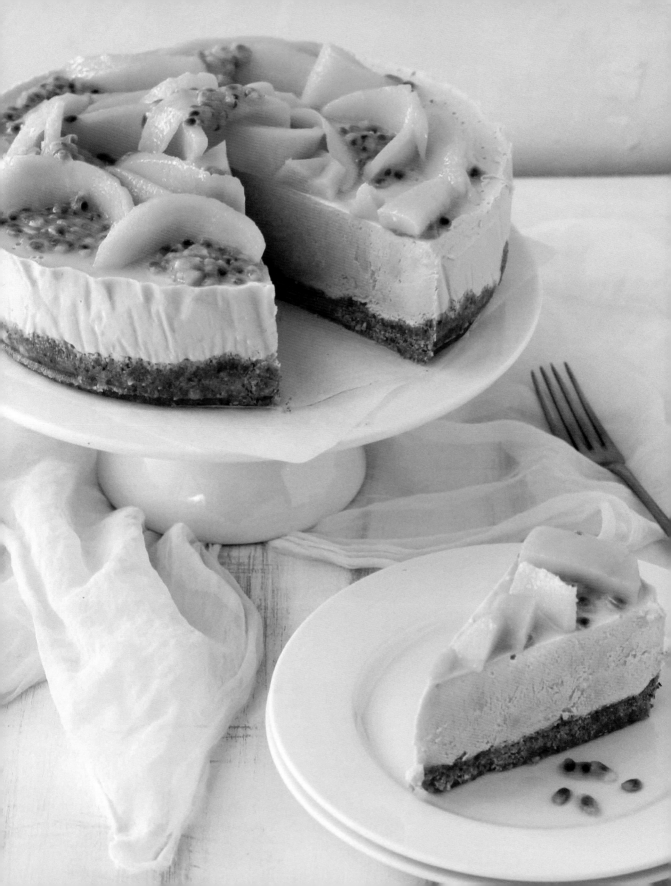

MANGO CHEESECAKE

PREPARATION: 20 MINUTES | SERVES 8–10

When gorgeous golden mangoes are in season I want to use them in as many ways as possible. Here's one of our favourite ways to enjoy this luscious fruit.

Crust
1 cup desiccated coconut
5 large Medjool dates, pitted
1 cup pecans

Filling
1 cup coconut cream
¼ cup maple or rice syrup
1 teaspoon agar-agar powder
2 tablespoons water
½ cup cashew nuts, soaked in water, rinsed well and drained
2 cups fresh mango pieces, plus 1 cup extra, to garnish
pinch of salt
½ teaspoon pure vanilla essence (vanilla extract)
juice of 1 small lemon
fruit of 2 large, sweet passionfruit, chopped, to garnish

To make the base, in a food processor grind the coconut and dates for 3–4 minutes, until the coconut starts to release its oil, then add the pecans and pulse briefly. Avoid pulsing for too long as it turns the mix to butter.

Transfer the mixture to a round 25-centimetre/10-inch glass baking dish and press down firmly and evenly. Place in the freezer while you prepare the filling.

To prepare the filling, combine the drained cashews, the 2 cups of mango (refrigerate the remaining mango in an airtight container; you won't need to use it for a while), salt, vanilla and lemon juice in a blender and blend until the mixture becomes smooth and creamy, about 1 minute.

Combine the coconut cream and syrup in a small saucepan and place over a medium heat, stirring, until it reaches a simmer. In a small jug or bowl, stir the agar-agar powder into the water until it dissolves completely and then stir this mixture into the hot coconut cream mixture. Increase the heat and bring the mixture to the boil for 1 minute, stirring constantly, then remove from the heat.

Add the warm coconut cream mixture from the saucepan to the blender and blend for 30 seconds, until it's silky smooth.

Remove the base from the freezer and pour the filling mixture onto the frozen crumb base. Refrigerate overnight or for at least 5–6 hours.

Remove the base and filling from the refrigerator and top with chopped mango and passionfruit. Slice with a warm knife to serve.

Variation
Use 1 tablespoon grated ginger in the crust for the cheesecake.

ICE-CREAM BASE

PREPARATION: 15 MINUTES | SERVES 8–10

Ice-cream truly is one of the most delicious treats we can share with those we love. Unfortunately, most commercial varieties are full of damaged fats, artificial flavourings, colourants and refined sugar. You don't have to deprive yourself, though, as these ice-cream recipes are made from real ingredients. If you find the mix too solid and not as fluffy as their commercial counterparts, you can churn the mixture in an ice-cream maker, achieving a similar texture to what you may be used to (you will need to double the ingredients). That's a little too time-consuming for me, so I do it the easiest way and simply freeze the whole mixture in a shallow glass dish or loaf dish when it's blended then stir it after 2–3 hours of freezing and enjoy slices of ice-cream.

1¼ cups cashew or
 macadamia nuts

1 cup coconut cream

¼ cup maple or rice syrup

1 tablespoon pure vanilla
 essence (vanilla extract)

¼ teaspoon salt

Combine all the ingredients in a blender and blend until very smooth and silky. Choose which of the following variations you'd like to make, then freeze the mixture in a glass loaf tin that will hold about 6 cups of liquid.

Variations

Hazelnut: 1 cup lightly roasted and skinned hazelnuts, or 1 bottle (240 grams/8 ounces) hazelnut butter, stirred through the ice-cream.

Mint: 2–4 drops mint essence (depending on how minty you want the ice-cream) added to the blender before blending.

Ginger: A few pieces of preserved ginger in syrup, finely chopped, and 1 teaspoon pure lemon essence stirred into the ice-cream base after blending.

Jam: ⅓ cup fruit juice sweetened jam, such as raspberry, strawberry, apricot or even marmalade, stirred into the base after blending.

Date: 4 large Medjool dates, pitted and soaked in coconut cream for a few hours and blended together until smooth and creamy, stirred into the ice-cream base before freezing.

Coffee: 1 tablespoon Swiss water-filtered, or carbon-dioxide extracted decaffeinated instant coffee granules dissolved in 3 tablespoons warmed coconut milk and stirred into 3 tablespoons of maple or rice syrup, stirred through the base before freezing. Reserve 2–3 tablespoons to drizzle over the ice-cream just before serving.

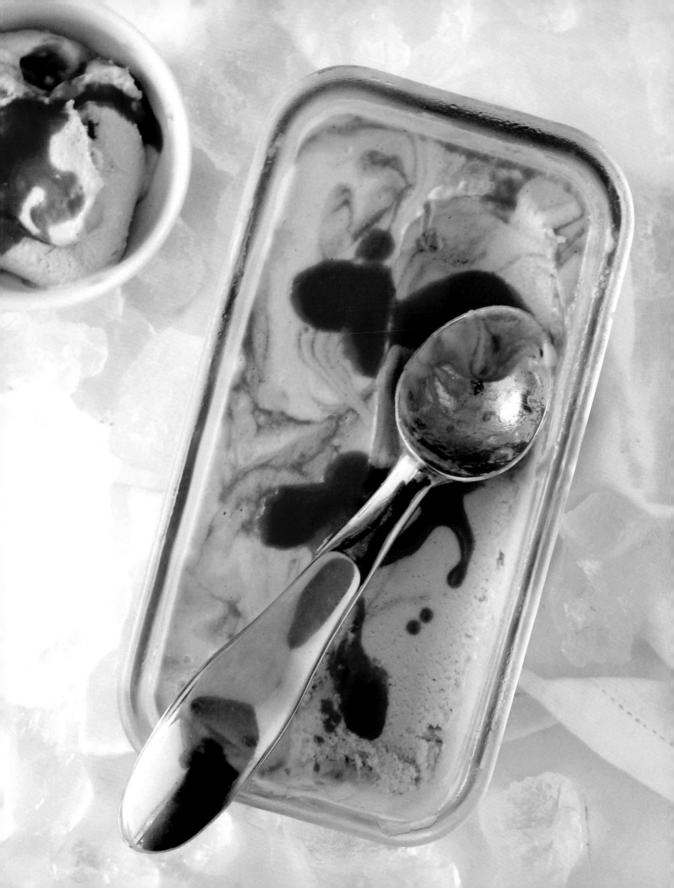

CHOC SAUCE TO SERVE WITH ICE-CREAM

PREPARATION: 10 MINUTES (PLUS 3 HOURS SOAKING TIME) | MAKES ¾ CUP

Store-bought chocolate sauces are full of refined sugar, damaged fats and other nasty compounds such as preservatives and artificial sweeteners. This option is nutrient-dense and much healthier.

6–7 Medjool dates, pitted

¾ cup macadamia, almond or hazelnut milk

1 teaspoon pure vanilla essence (vanilla extract)

¼ cup melted (25 grams/ 1 ounce) raw cacao butter

2 tablespoons raw cacao powder

In a bowl, cover the dates in your nut milk of choice, add the vanilla and leave to soak overnight or for 2–3 hours.

Melt the cacao butter in a saucepan over a low heat, and combine with the soaked dates and milk mixture. Transfer to a blender, add the cacao powder and blend until smooth and creamy.

SUPER-FAST CHOCOLATE SAUCE

PREPARATION: 5 MINUTES | MAKES ¾ CUP

This is a super-fast chocolate sauce that can be used over any ice-cream or over the cake on page 214. Either way, it's delicious!

¼ cup raw cacao powder

¼ cup maple or rice syrup

¼ cup coconut oil

½ teaspoon pure vanilla essence (vanilla extract)

Combine all the ingredients in a small saucepan and heat until bubbles form.

Remove from the heat and cool slightly before using.

Variation
Replace the cacao powder with carob powder for a different but still delicious flavour.

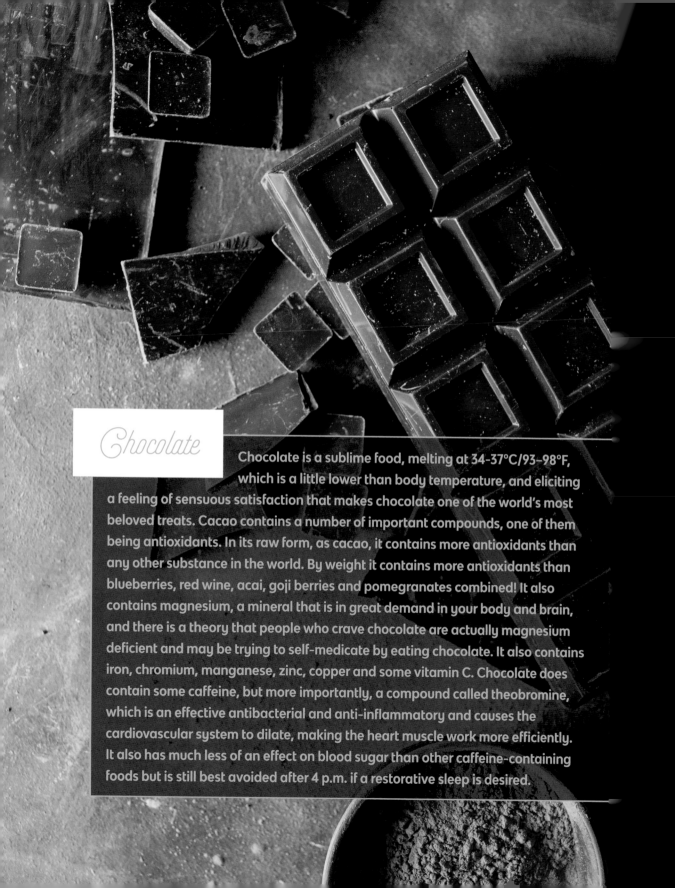

Chocolate

Chocolate is a sublime food, melting at 34-37°C/93-98°F, which is a little lower than body temperature, and eliciting a feeling of sensuous satisfaction that makes chocolate one of the world's most beloved treats. Cacao contains a number of important compounds, one of them being antioxidants. In its raw form, as cacao, it contains more antioxidants than any other substance in the world. By weight it contains more antioxidants than blueberries, red wine, acai, goji berries and pomegranates combined! It also contains magnesium, a mineral that is in great demand in your body and brain, and there is a theory that people who crave chocolate are actually magnesium deficient and may be trying to self-medicate by eating chocolate. It also contains iron, chromium, manganese, zinc, copper and some vitamin C. Chocolate does contain some caffeine, but more importantly, a compound called theobromine, which is an effective antibacterial and anti-inflammatory and causes the cardiovascular system to dilate, making the heart muscle work more efficiently. It also has much less of an effect on blood sugar than other caffeine-containing foods but is still best avoided after 4 p.m. if a restorative sleep is desired.

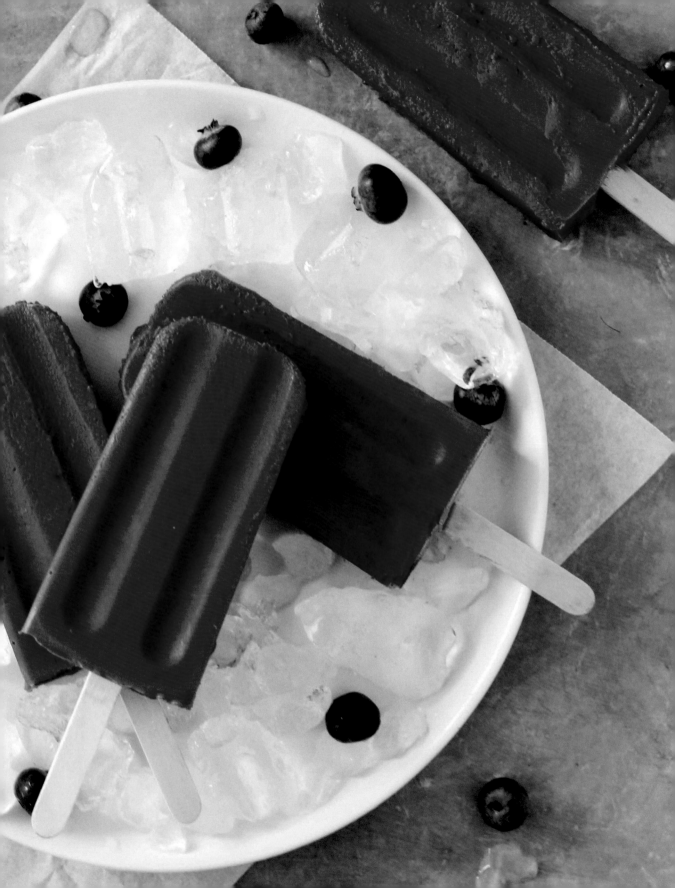

BERRY AND BEETROOT (BEET) ICE-CREAM/SORBET

PREPARATION: 10 MINUTES | SERVES 6–8

This is a very deep reddish-purplish ice-cream/sorbet and melts in the mouth with a delicious berry flavour. It is super-simple to make and apart from being delicious it's also impressive in terms of nutrient density. You can use popsicle moulds to freeze individual portions, or simply freeze in a glass loaf tin.

1 cup macadamia or cashew nuts, soaked in water for 2–3 hours, rinsed and drained well

¼ medium beetroot (beet), peeled and roughly chopped

⅛ cup coconut nectar, or maple or rice syrup

1 teaspoon pure vanilla essence (vanilla extract)

½ cup coconut cream

½ cup blueberries (frozen is fine)

½ cup pitted cherries (frozen is fine)

Combine all the ingredients in a blender and blend until smooth and creamy. Transfer to a glass container that can hold 6 cups of liquid and place in the freezer. Stir the mixture every hour until it has frozen. (Alternatively, freeze the mixture in an ice-cream machine according to the instructions.)

Remove from the freezer half an hour before serving to soften slightly.

Variation

Serve with fresh orange rind and a squeeze of fresh orange juice.

Tip

If you have a very powerful food processor or blender you can turn frozen fruit such as mangoes, bananas, pineapple, watermelon and berries of any variety into a sorbet in a few minutes. Simply add a few cups of frozen fruit and a little coconut milk to the food processor and blend on high until the mixture turns into a soft sorbet-like mixture.
Serve immediately.

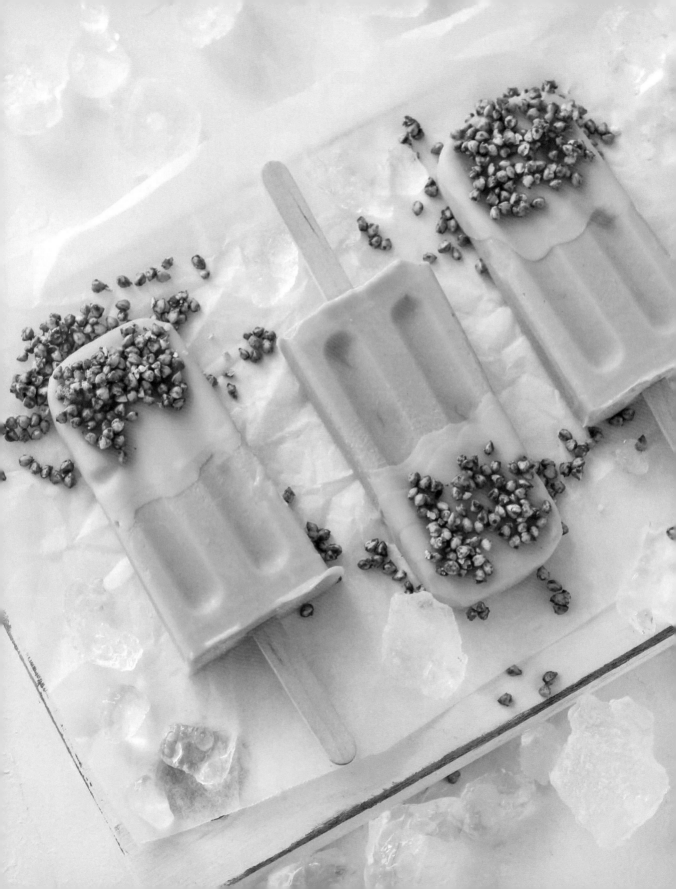

MANGO ICE-CREAM

PREPARATION: 10 MINUTES | SERVES 6–8

Mangoes are a summertime fruit, so it's the perfect time to make mango ice-cream. This is a very simple recipe to make, because you simply combine all the ingredients, practise patience overnight, and wake up to delicious, golden mango ice-cream. You can use popsicle moulds to freeze in individual portions, but you don't have to — it's perfectly fine frozen in a glass container too.

2 cups mango flesh, fresh or frozen

½ cup cashew nuts, soaked in water for 2–3 hours, rinsed and drained well

¼ cup coconut cream

2 tablespoons coconut nectar

2 teaspoons lemon juice

pinch of salt

1 teaspoon pure vanilla essence (vanilla extract)

Combine all the ingredients in a blender and blend until they form a smooth and silky cream. Transfer the mixture to either popsicle moulds or a glass container that can hold 6 cups of liquid. Freeze overnight.

If you are using a glass container, remove about 10 minutes before you plan to serve the ice-cream, because it needs to thaw slightly. If you make popsicles, dip the bottom into some plain white chocolate (see the recipe on page 184) and immediately dip into some buckwheat nibbles or roughly chopped almonds (see page 28).

Mangoes

There are more than 2500 known varieties of mangoes. They originated in the East Indies and Malaysia, being mentioned in Indian legends from 2000 BC, where they have been cultivated for more than 4000 years. They are related to cashew nuts. Traders in the 19th century introduced them to the West Indies, Africa and South America, but they are now grown throughout the Tropics, from the Caribbean to Africa and Australia. When they are smooth and hairless, mangoes are one of the most delicious fruits, but some varieties have hairy flesh. Their nutrient content is highest when they are ripe and their colour is deep yellow or orange. They are a valuable source of the antioxidants vitamin A and C, as well as vitamin K, and also contain some B vitamins, along with the minerals calcium, magnesium, phosphorus, potassium and zinc and plenty of fibre. They also contain a variety of other polyphenols, which act as antioxidants, such as zeaxanthin, which contribute to eye and brain health.

SPICED CHRISTMAS ICE-CREAM

PREPARATION TIME: 25 MINUTES (PLUS SOAKING TIME) | SERVES 15–20

This is a raw, dairy-free, refined-sugar-free dessert that is simple to make and super-tasty. A good friend designed a version of this ice-cream many years ago and I've changed it over the years because I enjoy the addition of coconut cream and orange essence. It is the perfect end to the large Christmas meal that most people indulge in during end-of-year festivities, and is a refreshingly cool and spicy alternative to the traditional hot Christmas pudding — especially for those of us who live in warm climates. Enjoy!

Fruit filling

⅓ cup seedless sultanas or raisins

⅓ cup dried Turkish apricots, thinly sliced

⅓ cup (6–7) small dates, or 3–4 large Medjool dates, pitted and thinly sliced

juice of 1 large orange, rind removed

Ice-cream

1 cup cashew nuts soaked in water for 2–3 hours, rinsed and drained well

1 cup coconut cream

1 large ripe banana, peeled and roughly chopped

½ teaspoon pure vanilla essence (vanilla extract)

rind of 1 large orange

1 heaped teaspoon ground cinnamon, plus extra, to serve

½ heaped teaspoon mixed spice

large pinch nutmeg

pinch of salt

To prepare the fruit filling, soak the sultanas or raisins, apricots and dates in the orange juice while you prepare the rest of the ice-cream.

To make the ice-cream, combine the cashew nuts, coconut cream, banana, vanilla, orange rind, cinnamon, mixed spice, nutmeg and salt in a blender, and blend until smooth. Add the fruit-and-juice mixture and pulse once or twice, quickly, to slightly break up the fruit but not completely.

Pour the whole mixture into a glass container that can hold 6 cups of liquid, and freeze.

Remove the ice-cream from the freezer about 15 minutes before you plan to serve the dessert to soften it slightly. Sprinkle each serve with a pinch of cinnamon.

Variation
Add 1 cup chopped macadamia nuts or almonds to the mixture for a nutty version.

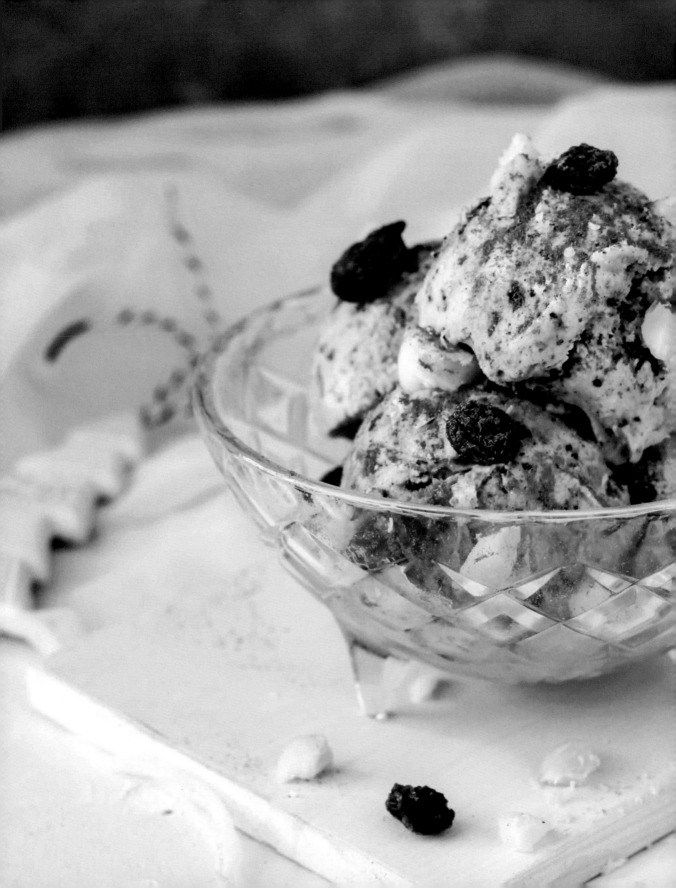

THREE-IN-ONE DARK CHOCOLATE ICE-CREAM, MOUSSE OR SAUCE

PREPARATION: 15 MINUTES | SERVES 6–8 | MAKES 3 CUPS

This is a very versatile recipe — you can use it as a chocolate sauce poured over one of the ice-cream variations on page 198, set it in the fridge as a mousse, or freeze it using an ice-cream machine as a third delicious variation. Quite by accident I discovered that it made a delicious mousse, when I stored it in the refrigerator, planning to add it to my ice-cream machine the next day. By the next morning it had set into a wonderful mousse. If you make it as an ice-cream be sure to soften it slightly before serving. If you have a very powerful blender you can simply combine all the ingredients and blend on high; otherwise, melting the chocolate separately as in step one below is necessary.

4 tablespoons raw cacao powder

150 grams (5 ounces) dairy-free, organic, unrefined sugar, 70 per cent dark chocolate

½ teaspoon pure vanilla essence (vanilla extract)

¼ cup coconut nectar, or rice or maple syrup

pinch salt

1½ cups cashew or macadamia nuts

1½ cups coconut cream

Combine the cacao powder, chocolate, vanilla, nectar or syrup and salt in a large bowl and place over a saucepan that contains water simmering over a low heat. Once the chocolate has melted, stir briefly, remove the mixture from the heat and allow it to cool to room temperature.

Meanwhile, combine the cashews and coconut cream in a blender and blend until smooth and silky. Add the cooled chocolate mixture and blend until very smooth. You can serve this as a chocolate sauce at this stage.

Transfer the mixture to a glass container that holds 6 cups of liquid, with an airtight lid, and refrigerate for at least 2–3 hours.

Either serve as mousse or transfer the chilled mixture to the freezer. Stir the mixture every hour until it has frozen. (Alternatively, freeze the mixture in an ice-cream machine according to the instructions.)

To serve as ice-cream, allow half an hour to thaw slightly before serving, and either slice it or scoop it out, serving with fresh berries and a dusting of cinnamon.

Variation
Combine 1 cup peanut butter with ¼ cup maple syrup and 1 teaspoon salt flakes. Add spoonfuls of this mixture to the chocolate mixture after you have poured it into a dish to either refrigerate for use as mousse, or freeze for ice-cream. This combines beautifully with the chocolate mixture to make an unforgettable dessert.

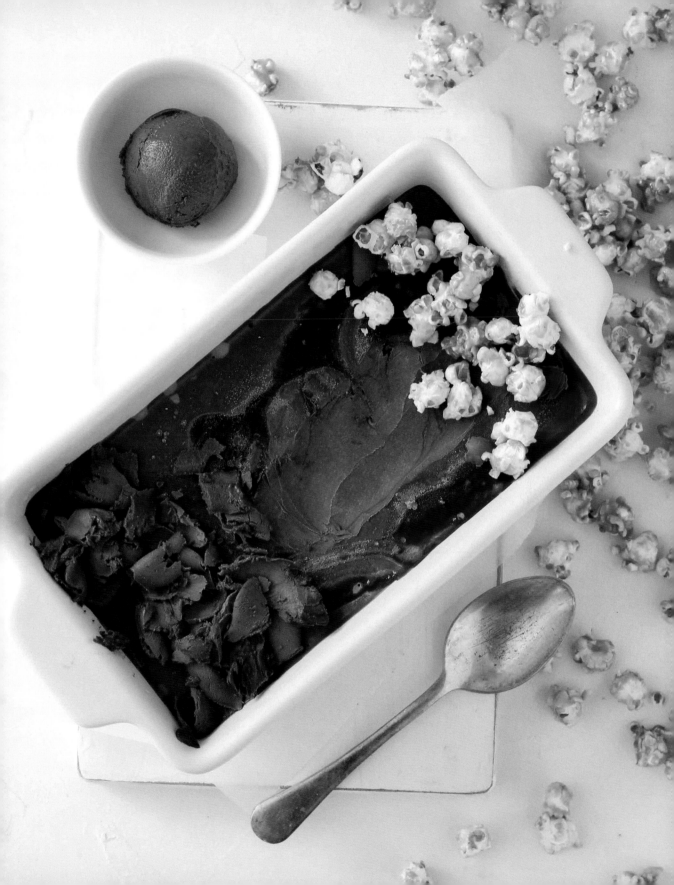

CARAMEL POPCORN (PICTURED P. 209.)

PREPARATION: 10 MINUTES | SERVES 8–10

This is a firm favourite and one I served at birthday parties for my children for many, many years — and watched as the adults devoured it too! Now my children make their own popcorn using a hot air popcorn maker, which is safe and very simple to use. This recipe is very simple to make and far healthier than the refined-sugar and additive-laden varieties available in-store.

10 cups popped popcorn

⅓ cup coconut oil

¼ cup coconut nectar, or maple or rice syrup

½ teaspoon salt

½ teaspoon bicarbonate of soda (baking soda)

1 teaspoon pure vanilla essence (vanilla extract)

Preheat the oven to 90°C/195°F. Line a large shallow pan with baking paper.

Place the popped popcorn in a large bowl.

In a medium saucepan, combine the oil, nectar or syrup and salt. Place over high heat and bring to the boil, then turn the heat off.

Remove from the heat and stir in the bicarbonate of soda and vanilla — the mixture will froth up. Pour over the popped popcorn and stir carefully, aiming to coat each popcorn piece.

Pour the coated popcorn into the lined pan and bake for 8–10 minutes, until light golden.

Turn off the oven. Stir and leave the popcorn in the oven with the door open for 5 minutes, then remove from the oven and allow to cool.

Variations

Sprinkle some chopped almonds over the popcorn after coating with the caramel sauce and then bake as above.

Drizzle some melted dark chocolate over the popcorn after it has cooled to make this treat even more delicious.

Savoury popcorn is now our favoured option — simply sprinkle some herb salt and olive oil over the popped popcorn and enjoy as is.

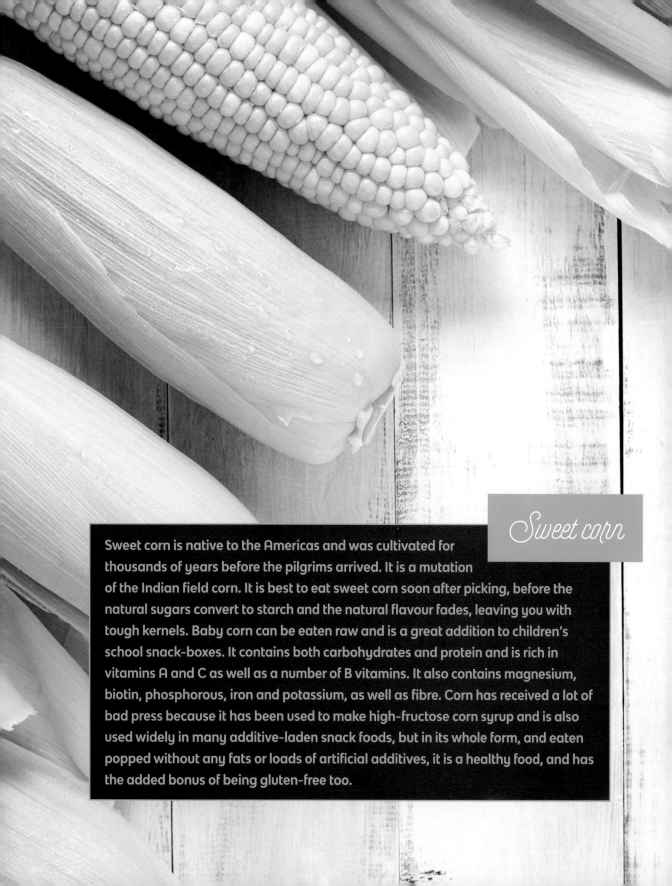

Sweet corn

Sweet corn is native to the Americas and was cultivated for thousands of years before the pilgrims arrived. It is a mutation of the Indian field corn. It is best to eat sweet corn soon after picking, before the natural sugars convert to starch and the natural flavour fades, leaving you with tough kernels. Baby corn can be eaten raw and is a great addition to children's school snack-boxes. It contains both carbohydrates and protein and is rich in vitamins A and C as well as a number of B vitamins. It also contains magnesium, biotin, phosphorous, iron and potassium, as well as fibre. Corn has received a lot of bad press because it has been used to make high-fructose corn syrup and is also used widely in many additive-laden snack foods, but in its whole form, and eaten popped without any fats or loads of artificial additives, it is a healthy food, and has the added bonus of being gluten-free too.

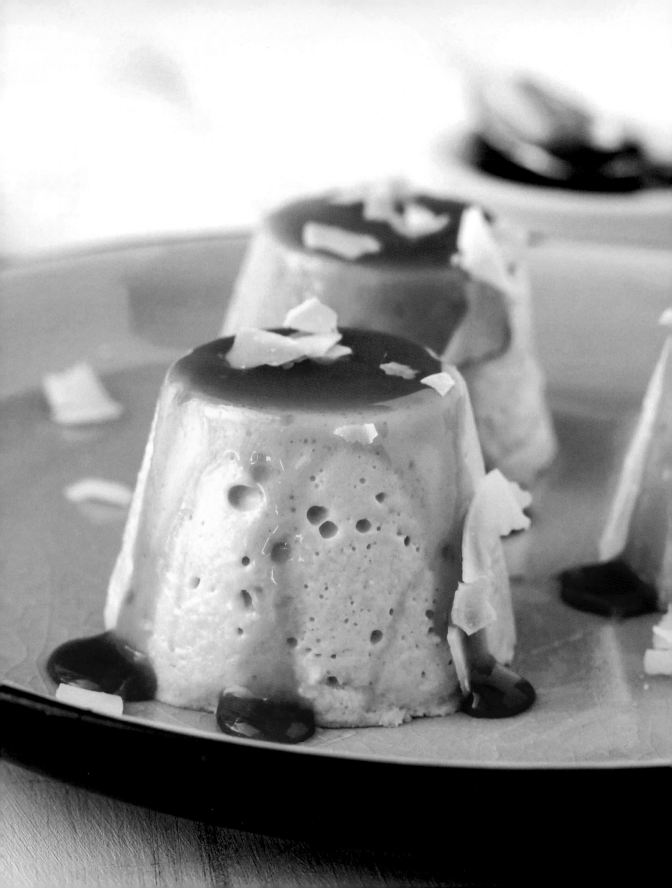

COCONUT AND BANANA CUSTARDS

PREPARATION: 20 MINUTES | MAKES 8 SMALL CUSTARDS

Simple to make, sublime and smooth to taste, without the dairy products and refined sugar that most custard desserts contain. You can sprinkle a few cubes of peeled mango, sliced strawberries or blueberries over each custard before serving, and a small teaspoon of maple syrup to make it look pretty. A sprinkling of cinnamon over the top adds to the flavour. Enjoy!

2 cups coconut cream

¼ cup coconut nectar, or maple or rice syrup

1 large banana

1 tablespoon pure vanilla essence (vanilla extract)

1 teaspoon agar-agar powder

Combine all the ingredients in a blender and blend until smooth. Transfer the mixture to a small saucepan and bring to the boil, then reduce the heat and simmer, stirring, for 4–5 minutes until it thickens slightly.

Transfer the mixture to small moulds and allow to set in the refrigerator for a few hours.

Tip

Agar-agar is a seaweed-based gelling agent used as a vegetarian replacement for gelatin. As a rule of thumb, to thicken 1 cup of liquid, use 1 teaspoon of agar-agar powder, 1 tablespoon of agar-agar flaked or ½ an agar-agar bar. Using the powder yields more consistent results. Substitute gelatin with the same amount of agar-agar powder. The solution you are trying to thicken with the agar-agar powder needs to be heated to boiling point and then allowed to simmer for about 5 minutes.

BITTER CHOCOLATE TART

PREPARATION: 15 MINUTES | SERVES 8–10

This is a simple tart to make, and it is very tasty if you enjoy a slightly bitter chocolate experience. You can make it the day before serving, but just be sure to drizzle a little warmed rice or maple syrup over it if it's going to stand in the fridge waiting to be served, because it tends to crack a little on top. If you don't have any almonds for the crust, simply use macadamia or cashew nuts. Or in a squeeze you can use coconut too. I like to serve this tart with raspberries that have been heated just until they wilt, or defrosted if frozen, and a drizzle of rice or maple syrup. Raspberries add a fresh, fruity lightness to the rich, dark decadent tart.

Crust
1 cup desiccated coconut

½ cup almonds

4 Medjool dates, pitted

2 tablespoons coconut oil

¼ teaspoon salt

⅛ teaspoon cayenne pepper

Filling
170 grams/6 ounces 70 per cent dark chocolate

1⅓ cups cashew nuts

3 large Medjool dates, pitted

1 cup coconut cream (saving a few teaspoons for swirling)

1 teaspoon pure vanilla essence (vanilla extract)

pinch of salt

To make the crust, combine the coconut, almonds, dates, coconut oil, salt and cayenne pepper in a food processor and blend until small-ish crumbs form.

Transfer the mixture to a round 20-centimetre/8-inch pie plate and press down firmly, either just along the bottom for a thicker base, or also up the side. Transfer to the freezer while you prepare the filling.

To make the filling, place the chocolate in a large bowl over a saucepan that contains water simmering over a low heat. Stir once or twice until it melts, which will take 3–4 minutes. Then remove from the heat and cool slightly. Transfer to a blender with the remaining ingredients and blend until the mixture is smooth and creamy.

Remove the crust from the freezer and pour the chocolate mixture over the crust. Swirl the leftover coconut cream over the filling, then refrigerate for a couple of hours before serving.

Variations
Add 2 drops peppermint essential oil.

Add 1 tablespoon psyllium husks to the base to add extra fibre.

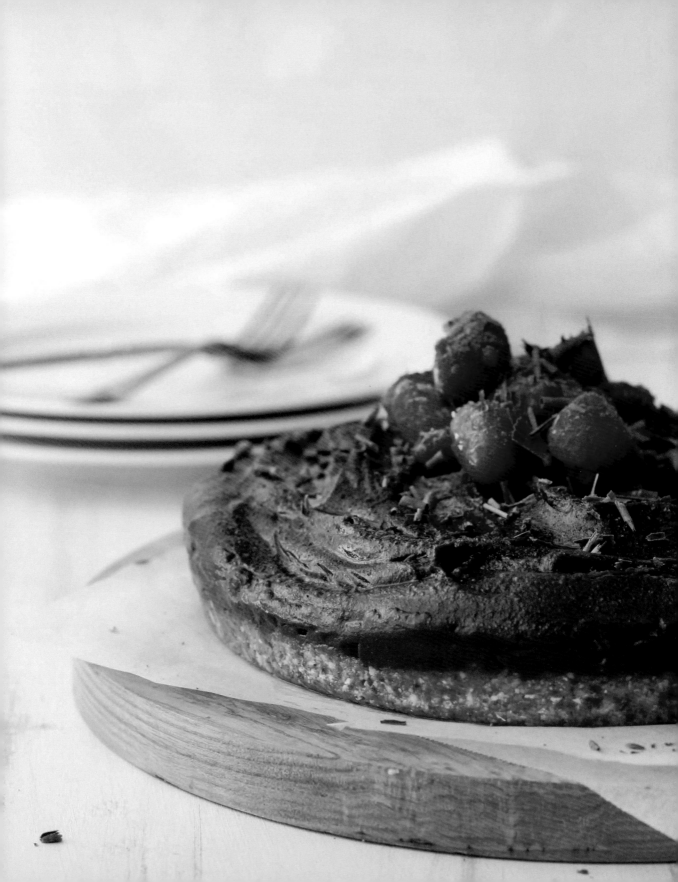

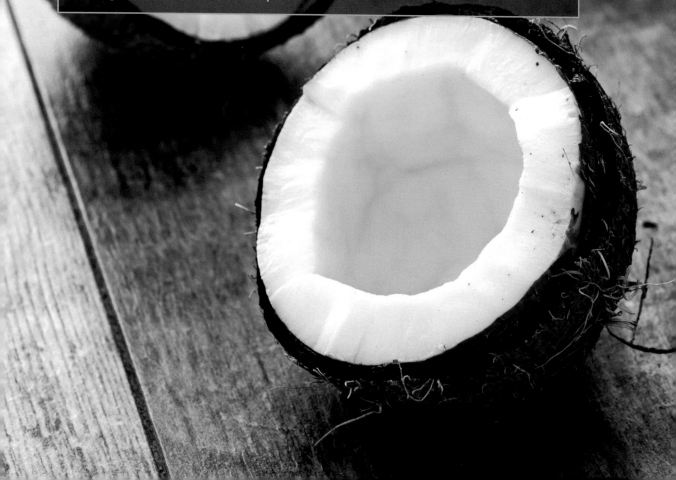

The coconut is versatile in terms of its uses and where it's happy to grow, from the Tropic of Cancer, north of the equator, to the Tropic of Capricorn, south of the equator. It is believed that this tree and its delicious fruit became as prolific as it is today firstly as a seed travelling from Pacific Islands, on the eastern Indian oceans, and then through humans transporting them through the tropics and beyond. Interestingly, coconuts are not a true nut, but actually the fruit of the coconut palm, and botanists classify coconuts as all three — fruits, nuts and seeds. They are high in a good form of saturated fat and also contain fibre, some B vitamins, as well as vitamin C, vitamin E, beta-carotene, iron, potassium and phosphorous. They contain a special type of fat, called Medium Chain Triglycerides (MCTs), which are antimicrobial, antiviral and antibacterial in action, as well as being beneficial in increasing metabolic rate. Coconuts are also a good supply of fuel for the brain. Coconut oil is best to use when you want to heat oil for cooking, because it's a very stable oil and minimally damaged when heated for short periods of time.

GOLDEN COCONUT AND ALMOND COOKIES

PREPARATION: 10 MINUTES | MAKES 30

These cookies are very simple to make and are high in protein. They are not overly sweet and make a lovely simple, nutrient-dense snack.

½ cup quinoa flakes

½ cup millet flakes

½ cup amaranth flakes

1 cup desiccated coconut

½ cup almond meal (or whole almonds)

3 tablespoons coconut oil

4 tablespoons coconut nectar, or maple or rice syrup

1 teaspoon pure vanilla essence (vanilla extract)

½ teaspoon coarse sea salt

½ teaspoon baking powder

1 teaspoon psyllium husks

Preheat the oven to 170°C/340°F. Line a baking tray with baking paper.

Combine the quinoa, millet, amaranth, coconut and almond meal (or whole almonds) in a food processor and grind roughly for 2–3 minutes, until the mixture resembles fine breadcrumbs. If the almonds are whole you will need to scrape the bowl down a few times between processing. Add all the remaining ingredients and process until a soft ball forms.

Put the mixture onto a sheet of baking paper and form it into a log with your hands, then cut into equal slices (about 2.5 centimetres/1 inch), laying each on the prepared baking tray. Bake for 10–12 minutes, until lightly golden.

Remove from the oven and allow to cool before sampling and then storing refrigerated in an airtight glass container for up to 10 days.

Tip

When cookies are made without damaged, shelf-stable fats, lots of refined sugar and nasty additives, they tend to get soft at normal room temperature. I therefore store all my cookies in the refrigerator where they stay crisp and fresh. I also prefer to make cookie baking as simple as possible, which is why I transform the mixture into a 'roll' and simply slice off even-sized discs to bake. However, feel free to shape these cookies into circles.

DARK CHOCOLATE COCONUT COOKIES

PREPARATION TIME: 15 MINUTES, PLUS 10 MINUTES BAKING TIME | MAKES ABOUT 30

When I was young I enjoyed a similar type of store-bought cookie, and I decided to transform it to a healthier version — and it tastes identical. They are simple to make and you can easily make a double quantity of dough, and roll half of the mixture into a waxed sheet of paper and store it in the freezer to make freshly baked cookies when you need a batch. You can leave the melted chocolate off them if you want to, but it adds to the chocolatey experience.

Cookies

¾ cup gluten-free flour 2 (see recipe on page 33)

¼ cup brown rice flour

1 teaspoon gluten-free baking powder

½ teaspoon bicarbonate of soda (baking soda)

3 tablespoons raw cacao powder

¼ teaspoon salt

¼ teaspoon pure vanilla essence (vanilla extract)

1 cup desiccated coconut

½ cup maple syrup or coconut nectar

½ cup coconut oil

Topping

100 grams/3½ ounces dairy-free, 70 per cent dark chocolate, or ½ cup chopped, melted

Preheat the oven to 160°C/320°F. Line a baking tray with baking paper.

Combine all the cookie ingredients in a food processor and mix until a soft ball of dough forms.

Tip the mixture onto a sheet of baking paper and use the paper to roll the mixture into a log, then cut into equal slices (about 2.5 centimetres/1 inch), laying each on the prepared baking tray. Bake for 10–12 minutes.

Leave the cookies in the oven but turn the oven off and open the door.

To make the topping, place the chocolate in an oven-proof glass bowl and put it on the bottom shelf of the warm oven, where it will melt slowly over 5 minutes.

Lay a piece of baking paper on a large flat plate. When the chocolate has melted, remove the cookies and the chocolate from the oven. Dip half of each cookie into the chocolate and lay them on the prepared plate. Refrigerate until they are set.

Ensure you store these cookies in an airtight glass container, because humidity will soften them.

Variations

Let the chocolate harden a little and then sandwich two cookies together with the melted chocolate.

Replace half the coconut oil with ½ cup peanut butter, and roll the chocolate log in ½ cup roughly chopped peanuts before slicing into cookies to bake.

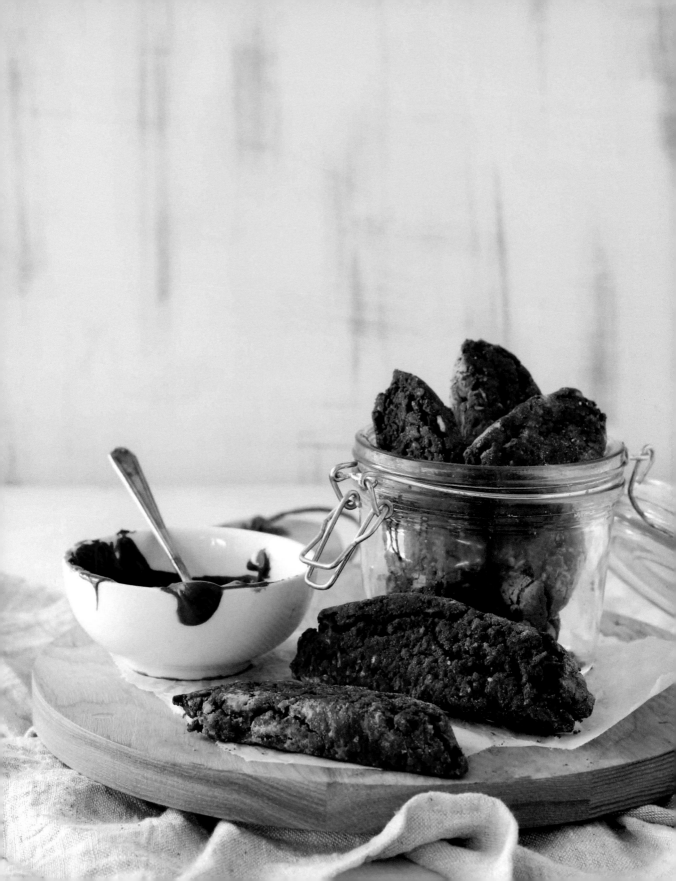

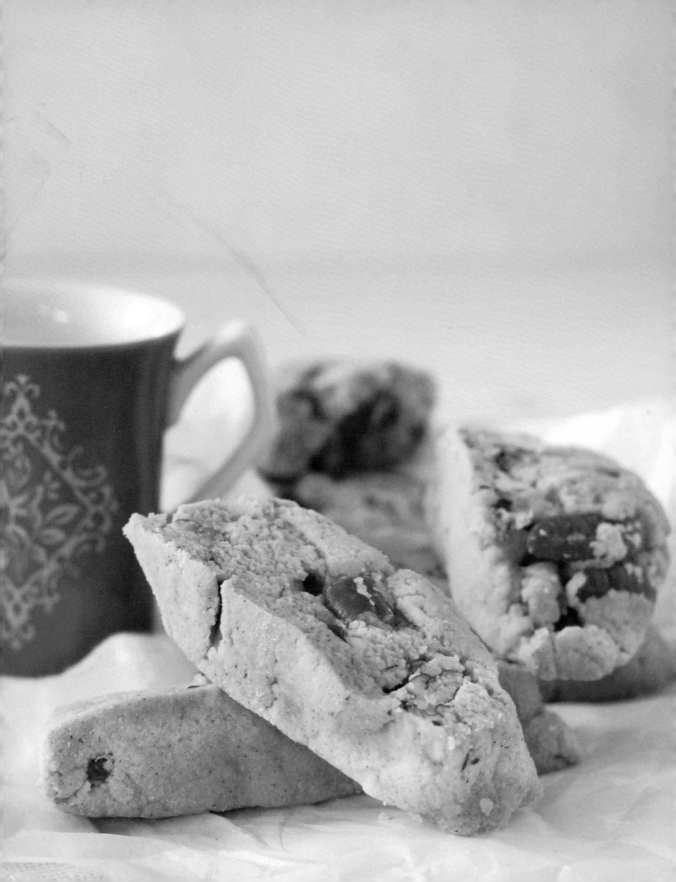

CRISP ORANGE AND SPICE COOKIES

PREPARATION: 15 MINUTES | MAKES 30

The Dutch have made deliciously crisp, spicy cookies for many hundreds of years. In this version I have replaced the eggs, milk, butter and sugar with healthier ingredients, leaving you with a cookie that is just as crispy and delicious. They never last long in our home!

2 cups gluten-free flour 2
  (see recipe on page 33)

2 teaspoons baking powder

1 heaped teaspoon ground
  cinnamon

¼ teaspoon ground ginger

¼ teaspoon ground nutmeg

¼ teaspoon ground cloves

pinch of salt

1 cup activated pecans,
  roughly chopped

½ cup coconut oil

½ cup coconut nectar or
  maple syrup

1 teaspoon orange rind, finely
  chopped, or ½ teaspoon
  orange essential oil

1 teaspoon lemon rind, finely
  chopped, or ½ teaspoon
  lemon essential oil

2 tablespoons rice flour

Preheat the oven to 160°C/320°F. Line a baking tray with baking paper.

In a large bowl, combine all the ingredients except for the rice flour, and mix well until a ball of dough forms.

Sprinkle the rice flour onto a sheet of baking paper and tip the ball onto this sheet. Use the paper to roll the mixture into a log and slice into 2-centimetre/¾-inch rounds, laying each on the prepared baking tray. Bake for 8–10 minutes until lightly golden in colour.

Turn the oven off, open the door and leave the cookies in the oven for 10 minutes. Remove from the oven and allow to cool completely before storing in a covered glass container.

Variations

Replace the pecans with almonds.

For a more decadent treat, dip half of each cookie into melted chocolate as per the dark chocolate coconut cookies (see recipe on page 218).

Pecan nuts

Pecan nuts are the only truly Native American nut and have a sweet, buttery taste. They grow wild throughout the south-eastern United States, and can live and bear edible seeds (nuts) for as long as 300 years. They are wonderful in green salads, grain dishes, muffins and as a topping for pancakes. They are very nutritious, containing mostly monounsaturated fats, along with protein, fibre, vitamins A,C,E,K and all the B vitamins except for B12, as well as calcium, iron, magnesium, manganese, potassium, phosphorous and zinc. They are the only natural food that American astronauts have taken into space. Remember, by soaking them in water, you increase their nutrient availability and brain benefits (see page 25).

PEANUT BUTTER AND CHOC-CHIP COOKIES

PREPARATION: 20 MINUTES | MAKES 24

This is a really simple cookie recipe with a delicious combined flavour of peanut butter and chocolate. Having all the ingredients in your pantry means that you can whip these up in no time.

1¾ cups gluten-free flour 2 (see recipe on page 33)

2 teaspoons baking powder

¼ cup rice flour

½ cup coconut oil

½ cup coarse peanut butter

¼ cup roughly chopped peanuts

⅓ cup maple or rice syrup

¼ teaspoon salt

¼ teaspoon pure vanilla essence (vanilla extract)

⅓ cup dairy-free 70 per cent dark chocolate chips

Preheat the oven to 150°C/300°F. Line a baking tray with baking paper.

Combine all the ingredients in food processor and pulse for 1 minute, until completely combined in a sticky ball.

Tip the mixture onto a sheet of baking paper and use the paper to roll the mixture into a log. Slice the log into 2-centimetre/¾-inch rounds, laying each on the prepared baking tray. Bake for 8–10 minutes, remove from the oven to cool, and then store in an airtight glass container in the refrigerator.

Variation

Replace the peanut butter with hazelnut butter, and replace the peanuts with roughly chopped hazelnuts.

Tip

If you don't have time to bake the cookies, or want to bake them fresh the next day, simply place the baking paper that contains the roll of cookie dough in a large zip-lock bag, seal, and place it in the refrigerator where it can lie flat. Remove from the refrigerator the next day and allow to thaw for about 10 minutes, then slice and bake as above.

Peanuts

Peanuts are legumes, not nuts, as they grow underground. They originated in South America 3500 years ago, where the Ancient Incas made a 'butter' paste with them. They are prone to a mould, namely aflatoxin, and unless organic contain high concentrations of pesticides. They are America's favourite snacking nut but half the crop becomes peanut butter. They are not healthy when covered in salt or sugar, damaged oils and additives. So choose plain organic peanuts and sugar-free butter to benefit from their protein content as well as B vitamins, iron, magnesium, manganese, potassium, selenium and zinc.

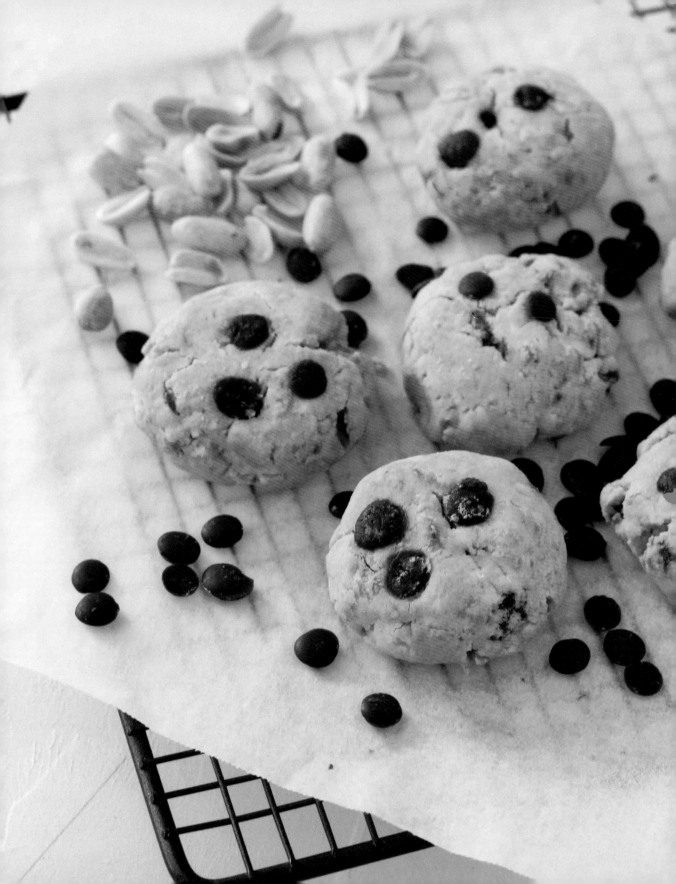

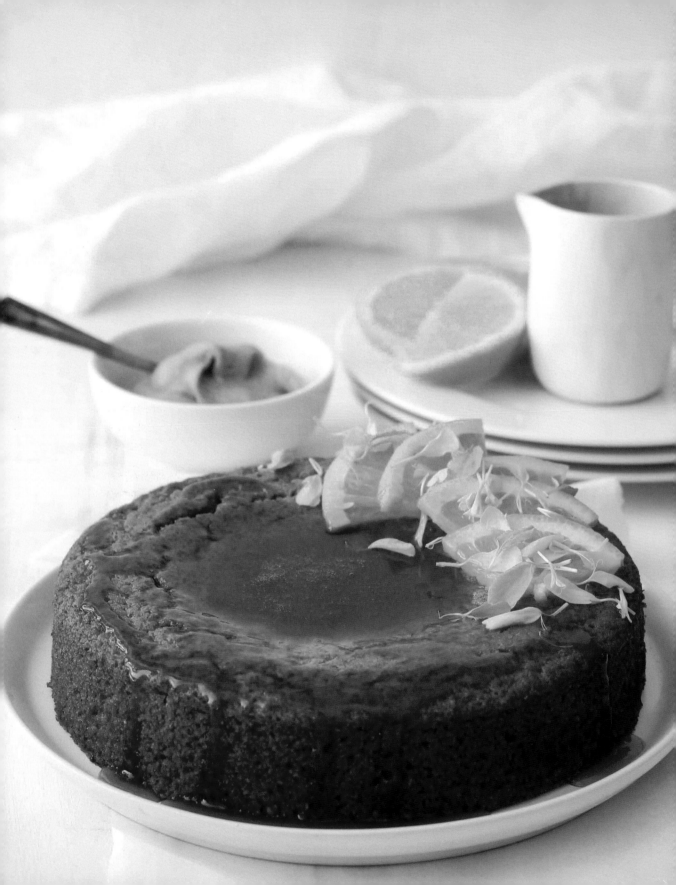

SPICE AND VANILLA GLUTEN-FREE CAKE

PREPARATION: 20 MINUTES (PLUS 25–30 MINUTES BAKING TIME) | SERVES 8–10

Creating a gluten-free, vegan cake isn't the easiest thing to do, and although this cake doesn't taste like a conventional sponge cake it is lovely and light and very nutrient-dense. You can also make cupcakes using this mixture — simply pour the mixture into a muffin tray, and bake for a little less time. You have to sift the gluten-free flour through a sieve because this will ensure a light cake, and make sure all the ingredients are at room temperature before assembling the cake. Follow the basic recipe below, then try the variations and toppings as great alternatives. It is also a great dessert with a dollop of orange cashew nut cream and a spoonful of warmed berries. If you want to make a two-layer cake, double the recipe and use one of the sturdier toppings to spread between the two layers.

1 cup gluten-free flour 2 (see recipe on page 33)

½ cup almond meal

¼ teaspoon salt

¾ tablespoon baking powder

½ teaspoon psyllium husks

½ teaspoon ground cinnamon

¼ teaspoon ground nutmeg

¼ cup coconut oil

½ cup maple syrup

¾ cup rice or coconut milk blend

rind of 1 orange, or 5 drops pure essential orange oil

½ teaspoon pure vanilla essence (vanilla extract)

Preheat the oven to 180°C/355°F.

In a large bowl, combine the gluten-free flour, almond meal, salt, baking powder, psyllium, cinnamon and nutmeg.

Combine the remaining ingredients in a blender and blend on high for a few seconds, until well combined. Slowly add the wet ingredients to the dry and stir carefully to just combine. The mixture will be quite runny.

Pour the mixture into a round 18-centimetre/7-inch baking tin, and bake for 25–30 minutes, until the edges come away from the sides of the tin and the top comes up when pressed lightly with your finger.

Remove from the oven and spread with one of the spreads below or eat as is while it is slightly warm.

Variations

Orange sauce: Combine 1½ cups orange juice, ½ cup maple syrup and 2 tablespoons orange rind in a saucepan and bring to the boil for 5 minutes until the mixture has reduced. Pour over the cake after it has cooled for 15 minutes.

Sticky date: Soak 3 large pitted Medjool dates in ⅓ cup coconut cream and 1 teaspoon pure vanilla essence (vanilla extract) for 2–3 hours and then blend with ⅓ cup macadamia or cashew nuts until a thick cream is formed. You can leave the nuts out and only use the coconut cream for a thinner sauce.

ACKNOWLEDGEMENTS

Family ... for your honest opinions and enjoyment of my meals. For giving the majority of them the thumbs-up, and suggesting improvements for those that didn't quite hit the mark. Thank you for your love and support! And to Emma and Matthew — here's to having the 'manual' for your own meals as you step out into the world on your own!

Mom ... for being the first one to introduce me to salads and sprouts looooong before they were trendy and became fashionable on social media. I am so grateful for your love and support!

Friends ... you know who you are. Those who popped in while I was experimenting, and those who requested recipes, and those who stood with me while I tossed, cooked and 'played' with food. Thank you to each and every one of you for your support — from near and far!

The Exisle team ... who once again made the journey from idea to complete book simple and clear! Thank you for your time and effort in making the experience as seamless as possible!

Vanessa ... thank you for your patience and clever creativity in making the food come alive, and helping me cope with transporting food on very hot days and working to tight deadlines!

REFERENCES

Aiello LC. 'Brains and guts in human evolution: The expensive tissue hypothesis*.' *Brazilian Journal of Genetics*. 1 Mar 1997; 20(1).

Baranski M, Srednicka-Tober D, Volakakis N, Seal C, Sanderson R, Stewart GB, et al. 'Higher antioxidant and lower cadmium concentrations and lower incidence of pesticide residues in organically grown crops: A systematic literature review and meta-analyses.' *The British Journal of Nutrition*. 14 Sep 2014;112(5):794-811.

www.businessinsider.com/countries-largest-antidepressant-drug-users-2016-2/?r=AU&IR=T [cited 15 December 2016]

Carmody RN, Wrangham RW. 'Cooking and the human commitment to a high-quality diet.' Cold Spring Harbour Symposium on Quantitative Biology. 2009;74:427-34.

Isler K, Van Schaik CP. 'How humans evolved large brains: Comparative evidence.' *Evolutionary Anthropology*. 2014 Mar-Apr;23(2):65-75.

Lemmens L, Van Buggenhout S, Van Loey AM, Hendrickx ME. 'Particle size reduction leading to cell wall rupture is more important for the beta-carotene bioaccessibility of raw compared to thermally processed carrots.' *Journal of Agricultural and Food Chemistry*. 22 Dec 2010;58(24):12769-76.

Lim SY, Kim EJ, Kim A, Lee HJ, Choi HJ, Yang SJ. 'Nutritional factors affecting mental health.' *Clinical Nutrition Research*. Jul 2016;5(3):143-52.

Link LB, Potter JD. 'Raw versus cooked vegetables and cancer risk.' *Cancer Epidemiology, Biomarkers and Prevention*. Sep 2004;13(9):1422-35.

Logan AC, Jacka FN. 'Nutritional psychiatry research: An emerging discipline and its intersection with global urbanization, environmental challenges and the evolutionary mismatch.' *Journal of Physiological Anthropology*. 2014;33:22.

McMartin SE, Jacka FN, Colman I. 'The association between fruit and vegetable consumption and mental health disorders: Evidence from five waves of a national survey of Canadians.' *Preventative Medicine*. 2013 3//;56(3–4):225-30.

Morris ZS, Wooding S, Grant J. 'The answer is 17 years, what is the question: Understanding time lags in translational research.' *Journal of the Royal Society of Medicine*. Dec 2011;104(12):510-20.

O'Neil A, Berk M, Itsiopoulos C, Castle D, Opie R, Pizzinga J, et al. 'A randomised, controlled trial of a dietary intervention for adults with major depression (the SMILES trial): study protocol.' *BioMed Central Psychiatry*. Randomized Controlled Trial Research Support, Non-U.S. Gov't. 2013;13:114.

O'Neil A, Quirk SE, Housden S, Brennan SL, Williams LJ, Pasco JA, et al. 'Relationship between diet and mental health in children and adolescents: A systematic review.' *American Journal of Public Health*. Oct 2014;104(10):e31-42.

Palermo M, Pellegrini N, Fogliano V. 'The effect of cooking on the phytochemical content of vegetables.' *Journal of the Science of Food and Agriculture*. Apr 2014;94(6):1057-70.

Rao TSS, Asha MR, Ramesh BN, Rao KSJ. 'Understanding nutrition, depression and mental illnesses.' *Indian Journal of Psychiatry*. Apr-Jun 2008;50(2):77-82.

Rucklidge JJ, Kaplan BJ. 'Nutrition and mental health.' *Clinical Psychological Science*. 1 November 2016;4(6):1082-4.

Rucklidge JJ, Kaplan BJ, Mulder RT. 'What if nutrients could treat mental illness?' *Australia New Zealand Journal of Psychiatry*. 2015;49(5):407-8.

Sarlio-Lähteenkorva S, Lahelma E, Roos E. 'Mental health and food habits among employed women and men.' *Appetite*. 2004 4//;42(2):151-6.

Sarris J, Logan AC, Akbaraly TN, Amminger GP, Balanzá-Martínez V, Freeman MP, et al. 'Nutritional medicine as mainstream in psychiatry.' *The Lancet Psychiatry*. 2015;2(3):271-4.

Thomas D. 'A study on the mineral depletion of the foods available to us as a nation over the period 1940 to 1991.' *Nutrition and Health*. 2003;17(2):85-115.

Thomas D. 'The mineral depletion of foods available to us as a nation (1940-2002) — a review of the 6th Edition of McCance and Widdowson.' *Nutrition and Health*. 2007;19(1-2):21-55.

www.time.com/growing-up-with-adhd/ [cited January 2017]

Worthington V. 'Nutritional quality of organic versus conventional fruits, vegetables, and grains.' *Journal of Alternative and Complementary Medicine*. Apr 2001;7(2):161-73.

RESOURCES

Check your local health food store and online for similar products in your area.

Blenders (including the Magic Bullet/NutriBullet)
www.vitamix.com
www.nutribullet.com

Ceramic nonstick frying pan
www.greenpan.com.au
www.neoflam.com.au/cookware

Ceres organics super grain penne — rice, amaranth and quinoa
www.ceres.co.nz/products/grocery/ceres-organics/
pasta-and-noodles/organic-super-grain-penne

Cobram Olive Oil
www.cobramestate.com.au

Coconut Magic
www.coconutmagic.com

Curry pastes
www.vivehealth.com.au/Organic-Natural-gluten-
Free-Curry-Pastes
www.watersteps.com.au/products/curry-pastes

Dona Cholita — fresh corn tortillas
www.donacholita.com.au

Explore Cuisine
www.explorecuisine.com/

Herbamare
I use a salt and herb product called 'Herbamare', which contains organic herbs and unrefined sea salt.
www.avogel.com.au/food/herbamare

Milks
I use Coco-Quench, a combination of organic coconut and rice milks for cereals, smoothies and baking purposes
www.pureharvest.com.au/products/coco-quench

Organic, Swiss water-filtered or carbon dioxide extracted decaffeinated instant coffee
www.republicaorganic.com.au/products/
decaffeinated-instant-coffee

Orgran gluten-free pasta
www.orgran.com

Power Superfoods
www.powersuperfoods.com.au/superfruits.html

Simply organic spices
www.simplyorganic.com

Teeccino dandelion caramel nut coffee alternative
www.teeccino.com/product/1046/Dandelion-
Caramel-Nut-11-Oz-Bag.html

Tio Pablo — instant corn masa mix
www.tiopablo.co.nz/product/masa-harina-800g

Udo's 369 Oil Blend
www.udoshealthproducts.com.au/
www.udoschoice.com/

Vanilla essence (vanilla extract)
www.au.iherb.com/pr/simply-organic-madagascar-
pure-vanilla-extract-farm-grown-4-fl-oz-118-
ml/31341
www.sunshinevanilla.com.au
www.greencaravan.com.au/product/spices-herbs-
condiments/vanilla-bean-powder-50g

Vegetable stock
www.australianorganicproducts.com.au/Marigold-
Organic-Yeast-Free-Veg-Bouillon-Cubes-p/
mar004.htm

Well & Good crusty bread mix — gluten-free
www.wellandgood.com.au/product/gluten-free-
crusty-bread-mix
See 'Extra Resources for *Feed Your Brain Cookbook*' at www.lighterbrighteryou.life

GENERAL INDEX

RECIPE INDEX